1

Advanced Myofascial Techniques

Shoulder, pelvis, leg and foot

Volume 1

Advanced Myofascial Techniques

Til Luchau

Foreword by
Robert Schleip

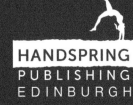

HANDSPRING
PUBLISHING
EDINBURGH

HANDSPRING PUBLISHING LIMITED

The Old Manse, Fountainhall,
Pencaitland, East Lothian
EH34 5EY, Scotland
Tel: +44 1875 341 859
Website: www.handspringpublishing.com

First published 2015 in the United Kingdom by Handspring Publishing
Copyright © Til Luchau 2015
Copyright in illustrations as indicated at the end of each chapter

ISBN 978-1-909-16-2

British Library Cataloguing in Publication Data
A catalogue record for this book is available from the British Library

Library of Congress Cataloguing in Publication Data
A catalog record for this book is available from the Library of Congress

Notice

Neither the Publisher nor the Author assumes any responsibility for any loss or injury and/or damage to persons or property arising out of or relating to any use of the material contained in this book. It is the responsibility of the treating practitioner, relying on independent expertise and knowledge of the patient, to determine the best treatment and method of application for the patient.

Commissioning Editor Sarena Wolfaard
Design direction and Cover design by Bruce Hogarth, KinesisCreative
Artwork by Primal Pictures unless otherwise indicated
Index by Aptara
Typeset by DSM Soft
Printed in Great Britain by Ashford Colour Press Ltd.

The
Publisher's
policy is to use
paper manufactured
from sustainable forests

Contents

Foreword

There have been numerous books written about myofascial approaches to hands-on manual therapy. Like this book, many of those come from the long lineage of fascial methodologies that include Ida Rolf's structural integration and its osteopathic influences, dating back to Andrew T. Still's writings on fascia from the late 1800s. And as this book does, many other books leverage our more recent learning about fascia to refine and enrich this long tradition.

However, the focus on a select set of common client complaints, and the provision of practical tools and suggestions for working practitioners to put into practice immediately, makes Til Luchau's book unique. Experienced practitioners will find thought-provoking concepts and details, with citations to relevant research, to help them take their knowledge and creativity to an even higher level. At the same time, newer practitioners will appreciate the clarity and accessibility of the verbal and visual instructions, as well as the step-by-step progression of the techniques.

However, clarity and simplicity should not be confused for a lack of substance or sophistication. During the more than 20 years that I have known Til Luchau as a colleague at the Rolf Institute of Structural Integration, I have learned an incredible amount from him while co-teaching numerous classes and exchanging information. His unique ability to offer valuable tools to both experienced and newer practitioners dates back to Til Luchau's early work at the Rolf Institute in Boulder, Colorado, USA. In the early 1990s, when Til Luchau was the Coordinator of that institute's Foundations of Rolfing Structural Integration program, he was charged with developing a curriculum to teach the fundamental manual therapy skills needed for structural integration. The resulting 'Skillful Touch' syllabus is still used (and being further developed) by the Rolf Institute's USA faculty today. A few years later, the Rolf Institute administration asked him to offer continuing education seminars for professionals in allied fields, introducing them to structural integration ideas to give them immediate tools to use, and inspire their further learning. His 'Advanced Myofascial Techniques' workshop series was immediately popular with bodyworkers, physical therapists, massage therapists, structural integration practitioners, chiropractors, and other hands-on specialists, and although official affiliation with the Rolf Institute ended amicably in 2010, today (in mid 2014) the Advanced Myofascial Techniques seminar series has several thousand alumni worldwide.

This book is therefore long overdue, and without a doubt will be welcomed by the many practitioners who have been exposed to Til Luchau's distinctive teaching, writing, videos, and broadcasts. It will be obvious to the reader that many years of evolutionary refinement underlie the ideas and instructions in this text.

This is not a Rolfing or even a structural integration text per se; not only is the Rolfing name trademarked, but Rolfing is much more than a set of techniques, and is less focused on client complaints than on the overall relationship of the body with gravity. Furthermore, there are many other influences in this book's material besides structural integration, including craniosacral therapy, osteopathic principles, orthopedic approaches, and the eclectic bodywork influences of Til's time practicing at the Esalen Institute in the 1980's.

There is more to any approach than its techniques. A quiet but pervasive point of view lies behind this book's anatomical language, compelling graphics, research citations, and detailed practical instruction. If you look closely, you'll see that Til Luchau's background in somatic and group psychology (having worked for many years as a somatic psychotherapist and group leader) comes through in a quiet, almost invisible way. This almost-hidden perspective emphasizes the human, interactive elements of hands-on work, and will find resonance with the many practitioners who feel that working *with* their clients or patients yields more satisfying results than working *on* them.

This attention to the interaction between practitioner and client, in combination with attention to the technical and physical sides of manual therapy, has parallels in our changing view of the connective tissue system itself. We are learning, for instance, that it isn't just fascia's interesting mechanical properties that account for its remarkable plasticity. It is becoming clear that fascia's innervation and resulting sensitivity also plays a very important role. The beneficial effects that manual therapists see may owe as much to this fascial sensitivity as to the fascia's purely physical properties (if not even more).

Of course the stunning images from Primal Pictures (and others) are a large part of this book's message. While we admire these images' intelligibility and beauty, let's remember that in the real body, myofascia is not neatly separated into discrete structures; it is fascia's often messy and complex interconnectedness that best characterizes it.

No book, no matter how lavishly illustrated or carefully worded, can substitute for the learning that happens in an in-person context. Many in this line of work learn through experiencing, feeling, and doing. Too often, books lead by thinking alone. This book's usefulness in a wide range of clinical and educational settings, and enduring value to practitioners, is that it includes all these dimensions.

Dr. biol.hum. Robert Schleip
Director, Fascia Research Group
Division of Neurophysiology
Ulm University, Germany

Preface

The ability to ease another's pain is meaningful in a way that few other things are. Pain cries for relief—biologically it functions to motivate the sufferer to stop something hurtful, or to seek respite. When someone in pain comes to us for help, we are much more than just practitioners of a therapeutic modality; we are, in that moment, fellow human beings, together with another person facing a pressing biological problem. When we can reduce the pain of those who come seeking our help, we are fulfilling a need that lies at the core of our species' biological and social functioning. Few things provide as much meaning and purpose.

Of course, our work is not just about relieving pain. Not everyone comes to us because of pain. Sometimes, we are most effective when we raise our clients' or patients' level of functioning to extend it beyond the simple absence of pain or dysfunction. And even when it seems like we can't ease the physical pain of those who have come to us for relief, our work can still be useful in many profound ways; in fact, it is in these moments that both our mastery and our humanness are most needed.

Still, when we can help relieve pain, we should. The techniques described in these books represent some of the most effective ways that I have found for doing this. They do not represent the whole story by any means—there are many, many other ways of accomplishing similar goals, and there are numerous techniques that did not make it into the text, simply because they did not lend themselves to written description.

The techniques described here are taken from the body of work taught in Advanced-Trainings.com's Advanced Myofascial Techniques' series of workshops and video courses. In its principal and specialty courses, this seminar series presents a comprehensive system for working with the entire body, currently encompassing over 40 session sequences and more than 350 techniques, tests, and procedures. The techniques chosen for this volume (focusing on conditions of the appendages), as well as those selected for the next one (which will include techniques for spine, rib, head, and neck complaints) represent a set of effective and accessible tools for some of the most common client complaints. While they can be used as stand-alone techniques, I recommend learning more about this approach through the other available training formats and media (many of which are free and online).

Goals of the work

Paradoxically, even though the techniques described here are often very effective in addressing pain, relief from pain is only a secondary benefit of this way of working. Our two primary goals are:

1. Increase options for movement;
2. Refine the proprioceptive sense.

The first goal (increase options for movement) includes all magnitudes of movement and mobility, ranging from subtle micromovement pulsations to gross range of movement. This means that we employ the entire spectrum of depth and pressure with our touch. Often, our techniques use direct pressure to affect a gross movement change. Sometimes, larger mobility isn't possible until the smaller, subtler intrinsic motions (such as movements of craniosacral therapy, visceral manipulation, and so on) are also addressed. Accordingly, you will see both deep, direct touch, and subtle receptive touch used in the techniques here.

The second goal (refine proprioception) implies that we want our clients to feel their bodies in new and enhanced ways as a result of our work. 'Proprioception' includes the sensations of one's own body position and movement, and our touch, pressure, and the movements we ask for can all evoke proprioceptive learning. Recent research into the mechanisms of myofascial change suggests that there is a much larger role for proprioception than has been assumed in the past (discussed further in Chapter 2, *Understanding Fascial Change*). When this body sense is awakened, it lays the groundwork for finer, more efficient movement coordination. It also paves the way for many other benefits, such as the development of more sustainable in-the-moment postural choices.

Secondary to these main goals, these techniques bring about other benefits. Pain, athletic performance, well-being, etc, all tend to improve when our two primary goals are addressed. However, less pain, improved performance, and any other benefits are the end results; the means to those ends are simply to increase our clients' options for movement, and invite more refined proprioception.

Of course, other goals can be served by the techniques and tools described here. A structural integration practitioner might see applications for improving alignment and integration. Similarly, physical therapists, acupuncturists, massage therapists, rehabilitation specialists, and others will see ways to use these tools to serve their modalities' therapeutic goals. But using these two primary goals (more movement options and refined proprioception) as touchstones will help simplify, clarify, and focus each technique's purpose and application.

This book's assumptions

This book is intended for trained manual therapy practitioners in professional practice (such as structural integration practitioners, physical and physio- therapists, physical therapy assistants, body-workers, massage therapists, osteopaths, chiropractors, acupuncturists, and other hands-on practitioners). It is also appropriate for use by intermediate and advanced students of these disciplines who are using this text within a training context. Accordingly, this book assumes that the reader has familiarity with considerations and contraindications for deep hands-on work. Where particularly important, or where not obvious, these considerations are described in the text, but a basic level of training and knowledge is assumed.

These techniques are intended as tools to be used within the larger context of a session or series. Elements of this larger context might include interviewing, assessment, preparation, strategizing and sequencing, balancing, closing, and integration back into daily life. Each modality has its own ways of accomplishing these functions, and (although some discussion of sequencing is planned for volume two), I will assume that the reader has this training as well.

Books like this can serve to stimulate your imagination, innovation, and versatility. However, I assume that the reader will realize that you really cannot learn all you need to know about these techniques from a book. To some extent, video can help to round out the picture, and this book includes video links to many of the techniques described (with video of all techniques being available in the companion video sets). However, the most important aspects, which have to do with the kinesthetic and experiential realities of actual touch and sensation, can only be acquired through in-person mentoring and feedback, as well as by actually receiving and experiencing the work being described.

Of course, this book is just a starting point. As valuable as the methods and points described in this text are, there comes a point where better techniques and tricks just aren't the answer. Relieving pain can be relatively simple; however, when pain does not go away, our mastery and deeper humanness is called forth. It is then that we are faced with Austrian-born philosopher Marten Buber's dichotomy: we can either see others as objects (as "clients," "patients," or problems to be fixed), or as actual people—unique, multidimensional, sentient beings, just like ourselves.

Til Luchau
Boulder Colorado, 2014

Acknowledgements

Almost everyone knows that writing a book takes work. What isn't obvious is that a book takes many people's work.

A special thanks to my colleague, friend and mentor Dr. Robert Schleip for his encouragement, and for his inspiring example of continuing fascination, learning, facilitative leadership within our field, and beyond. Like an orchestral conductor, he brings out the best in those around him, and we all benefit from his talents.

Thanks to Leslie Young PhD, Editor-in-Chief at Massage & Bodywork Magazine, for featuring the ongoing Myofascial Techniques column, where many of these ideas first appeared. Her skilled team, including Darren Buford, Amy Klein, and others helped shape the first drafts of this material. Anne Williams and Brian Halterman at the Associated Bodywork & Massage Professionals (ABMP) played an important role by sponsoring and hosting the Myofascial Techniques webinar series.

I am grateful to Sarena Wolfaard, Andrew Stevenson, Bruce Hogarth at Handspring Publishing Limited, for their patience, persistence, flexibility, and collaborative spirit. Their dedication to quality, and passion for this field, has been a joy to work with.

My esteemed faculty colleagues at Advanced-Trainings.com have continually contributed ideas, critique, dialog, techniques, and inspiration. They include Larry Koliha, George Sullivan, Chris Pohowsky, Ellyn Vandenberg, Bethany Ward, as well as many dedicated and skilled teaching assistants and students around the world that are too numerous to list, but just as deserving of acknowledgement.

Advanced-Trainings.com instructor Bethany Ward read every word I wrote, and made expert suggestions and corrections, often up against tight deadlines. Patrick Dorsey contributed countless hours towards the book's study guide questions, as did other question-writing interns. Thanks to Christina Galucci and Daniel Glick for their skilled editing and support as well.

Acknowledgements

Over 12 years ago, Primal Pictures' graphics first opened my eyes to the beauty and surprising learning that's possible when the body's anatomy can be viewed, rotated, and layered in three dimensions. Photographic models Erin Trunck, Fika O'talora, David Videon, and David Lowell, as well as photographers Kit Hedman and Rick Cummings all contributed to the aesthetics of this project. Heartfelt thanks to the many artists and researchers who licensed and generously gave re-use permissions for the images in this book. They are listed In the picture credits.

My mentors and colleagues at the Rolf Institute have of course been a profound influence on the material here. I am grateful to the influence and support of Jan Sultan, Pedro Prado, Thomas Myers, Art Riggs, Bibiana Badenes, Erik Dalton, and many others. For 30 years, my clients in my private practice have been some of my best teachers, as have the practitioners who bring their difficult supervision cases for our mutual learning.

Warm appreciation is due to the many people who generously extended indefatigable hospitality by helping provide quiet places to write this book: Anna Maria Gregorini in Zurich; Lynn Phillipon and Nikki Gillespie in southwestern Colorado; K'lea Andreas in Victor, Idaho; Robert Gajdoš in Prague; Paula Earp and the practitioner community in Fairbanks, Alaska; and many, many others.

And to my son Ansel Luchau, and especially my wife Loretta Carridan Luchau, who have patiently supported me in the long process of writing a first book. This book is lovingly dedicated to them.

Reviewers

Bibiana Badenes, P.T.
Physical Therapist, Certified Advanced Rolfer™, Certified Rolf Movement® Teacher; Director, Kinesis Center and Movement Therapy; President, BodyWisdom Foundation Spain
Benicasim, Spain.

Erik Dalton, Ph.D.
Certified Advanced Rolfer™; Author;
Executive Director, Freedom From Pain Institute
Oklahoma City, Oklahoma, United States.

Rachel Fairweather BA, LMT, AOS Massage Therapy, CQSW
Director, Jing Advanced Massage Training; Author
Brighton, United Kingdom.

Cheryl LoCicero, B.Sc. R.M.T
Certified Advanced Rolfer™, Certified Rolf Movement® Teacher, Fascial Integration: Structural-Visceral approaches
Consultant, Center for Complementary and Alternative Research and Education, University of Alberta
Edmonton, Alberta, Canada.

Budiman Minasny, Ph.D.
Researcher, University of Sydney
Sydney, Australia.

Peter B. Pruett, M.D.
Physician – Board Certified in Emergency Medicine
Delta County Memorial Hospital
United States Air Force Academy; University of Colorado, Denver
Hotchkiss, Colorado, United States.

Art Riggs
Certified Advanced Rolfer™; Author
Director, Art Riggs Deep Tissue and Manual Therapy Educational Systems
Berkeley, California, United States.

Susan G. Salvo, M.Ed., L.M.T.
Author – Educator – Massage Therapist
Elsevier Health Science; Louisiana Institute of Massage Therapy
Lake Charles, Louisiana, United States.

Robert Schleip, Ph.D. M.A.
Visiting Professor (IUCSAL)
Director, Fascia Research Group
Division of Neurophysiology, Ulm University
Ulm, Germany.

Bethany M. Ward, M.B.A., L.M.B.T.
Certified Advanced Rolfer™, Rolf Movement® Practitioner
Faculty, Rolf Institute® of Structural Integration
Advisor and Past President, Ida P. Rolf Research Foundation
Director, ActionPotential, Inc.
Durham, North Carolina.

Online Resources

Scan the code or visit http://advanced-trainings.com/amt1/ for supplementary online resources, including:

- Online video library
- Professional Continuing Education and CMA credit options
- Teacher and student classroom resources
- Free myofascial webinars
- Forum and social media links for questions and dialog about Advanced Myofascial Techniques
- Offers and discounts from Primal Pictures, Advanced-Trainings.com, and others mentioned in this book.

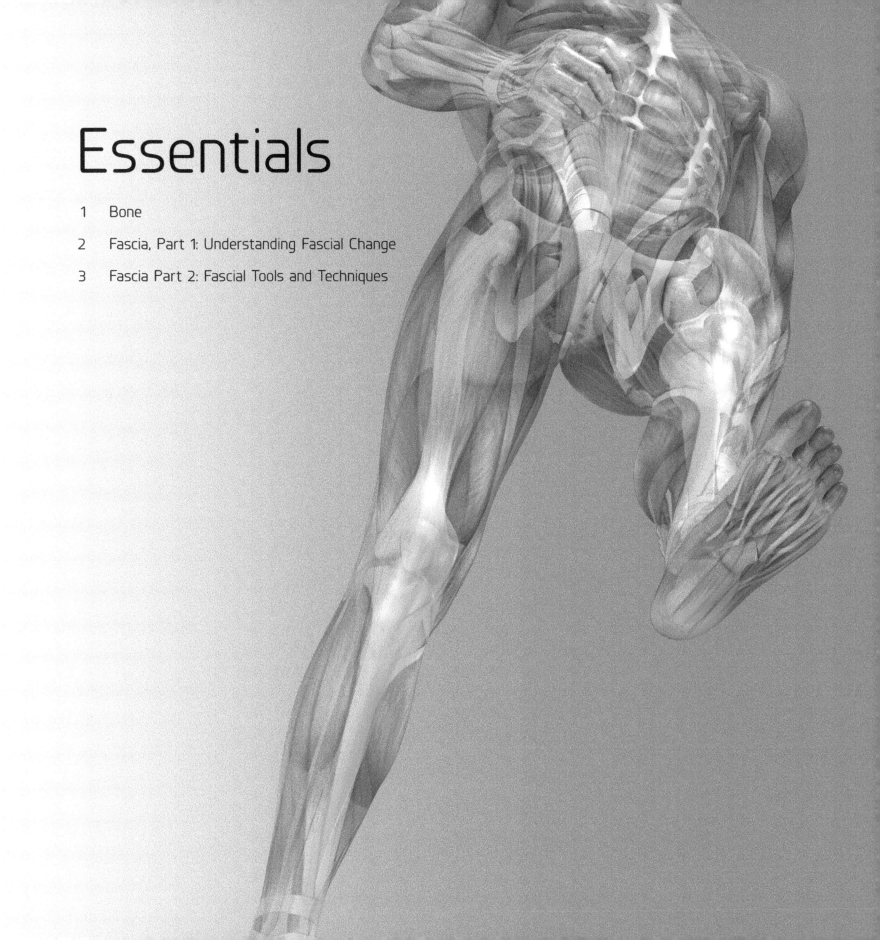

Essentials

Bone

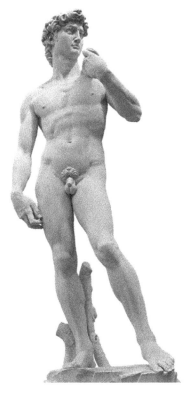

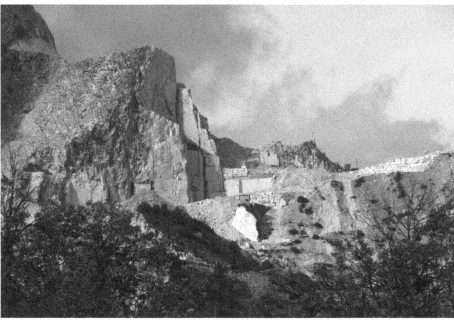

When Michelangelo was a young man, he petitioned the senior sculptor, Bertoldo di Giovanni, to accept him as his student. Legend says Bertoldo gave Michelangelo a prerequisite: "You want to carve marble?" the mentor said, "First, go work as a stonecutter in the marble quarry. Get to know marble."

"For how long?" asked Michelangelo who, although just a teenager, was already an accomplished painter.

"Two years in the quarry," said the sculptor. "Then, you can begin to sculpt."

Whether fact or legend, this story tells us about the value of getting to know our media – the actual materials and substances we work with – before we try to become artists or masters. Those of us who do hands-on work with the body need facility in many media. Examples include fascia and other connective tissues, skin, or muscle when we do structural or tissue work; or blood flow and muscular tension when we are performing classical massage. Likewise, our client's movement, coordination, and balance are our media when we are working functionally; energy and flow come into play in energetic modalities, and the client's autonomic state could be said to be our medium when our intent is to relax or calm. Each manual therapy modality is distinguished not only by what it aims to accomplish, but also by the media it works with to accomplish those ends.

Although we work with many other tissues and systems in our Advanced Myofascial Techniques trainings, we begin with bone in the same spirit that Michelangelo was asked to start in the quarry (Figures 1.1–1.3): to get to know the nature of one of the body's fundamental tissues. In this chapter, I will focus on bone as one of the primary mediums of our art.

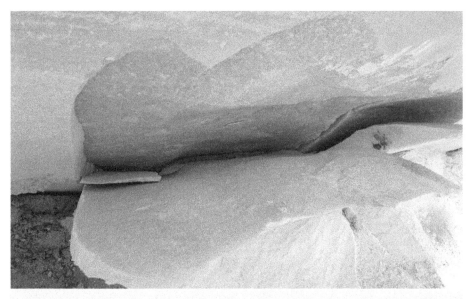

Figures 1.1/1.2/1.3

Michelangelo worked as a stonecutter before becoming a sculptor. David (Figure 1.1) was sculpted using marble (Figure 1.2) from Carrara quarry (Figure 1.3). Michelangelo began working on David in 1501 when he was 26 years old, less than 10 years after his studies with Bertoldo.

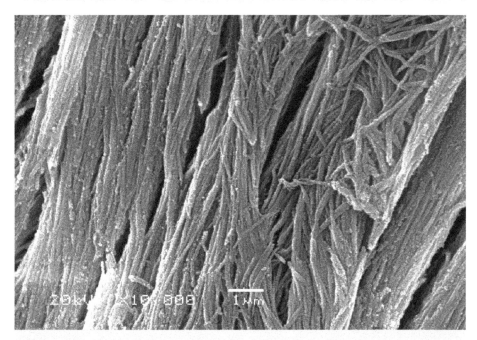

Figure 1.4

Electronic micrograph of mineralized collagen fibers in bone. Living bone is about 25% collagen, which adds flexibility. Naish, J. et al. Medical Sciences. Elsevier (2009).

In the embryo, bone arises from the mesoderm – the same tissue layer from which muscle and connective tissues, such as fascia, tendons and ligaments, form. Like these tissues, bone is composed of cells, fibers, and other components, all of which are embedded within a surrounding matrix. In bone, this matrix accounts for about half of the bone's weight, and it is largely composed of phosphate and calcium in a microcrystalline form called *hydroxylapatite*. Structurally, these apatite crystals are relatively weak by themselves – think of a piece of chalk. However, in the body, these mineral nanocrystals are molecularly linked and interwoven with thin, flexible, collagen fibers (1) (Figures 1.4 and 1.5), forming a fiber/matrix composite, analogous to fiberglass or bamboo (Figure 1.6). Bone's composite nanostructure of mineralized collagen fibrils keeps microscopic fractures from spreading, and adds surprising flexibility to the bones. Like synthetic fiber/matrix nanocomposites, it is also extremely strong – pound for pound, living bone is even stronger than cement.

Unlike cement, however, living bone has qualities that we do not usually associate with the dry, dead bones we know from skeletons in anatomy class (Figure 1.7). Living bones are up to one-third larger than dried bones, largely due to the water they contain when alive. They are also softer and more adaptable, just as a living starfish is soft and pliable when compared to a hard, brittle, dead specimen (Figure 1.8).

Living bones are also very sensitive. The periosteum, or fibrous "bone skin" surrounding bones is highly innervated (Figure 1.9). Its many mechanoreceptors help coordinate movement and balance by sensing the pull of the skeletal muscles where their tendons blend with the bone's periosteum at attachment sites. The articular ends of long bones are also particularly sensitive, which assists with proprioception and movement coordination. It has long been known that there are

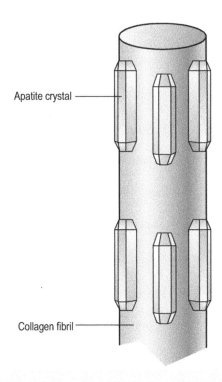

Figure 1.5

Bone's calcium is in the form of microcrystalline apatite, which binds to these collagen fibers, giving them far greater toughness than they would have alone.

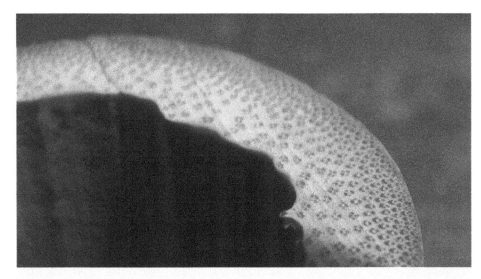

Figure 1.6

Like bone, bamboo is a fiber/matrix composite.

also numerous nerves inside the bones, such as the small myelinated nerve fibers that wind through the spongy trabeculae deep within cancellous or spongy bones (2). The nerves that are present within bone are one of the reasons why fractures and bone bruises can be so painful; however, this also means that your clients can literally feel your touch in their bones.

In Advanced-Trainings.com's Advanced Myofascial Techniques series, we use bone-focused techniques for three purposes: to feel for greater mobility, greater motility, or greater connection.

Feeling for Mobility

Mobility is defined as *the ability to be moved*. In our approach to hands-on work, our methods often focus on moving bones. This is not a chiropractic or osseous adjustment; rather, we use bones as levers or handles to assess, mobilize, and release the surrounding myofascia. When working for greater mobility, the practitioner's pressure is usually firm, as we are feeling for direct release of any shortened, tightened, or constricted connective tissue structures that limit the bones' mobility.

This passive movement of the bones is useful when preparing for deep connective tissue work, since it allows the practitioner to both assess and release gross movement restrictions at the articular level. However, we are not looking to indiscriminately increase the amount of gross movement at a joint; instead, we feel passive bony mobility and compare one joint against another or one direction against its complement, and we work specifically to free the more restricted aspect. This brings balance to the release.

Techniques that work with bony mobility also stimulate proprioceptive sensation at the very deepest levels, since the bones themselves have rich sensory innervation. Sensations produced by the work wake up and enliven the body sense,

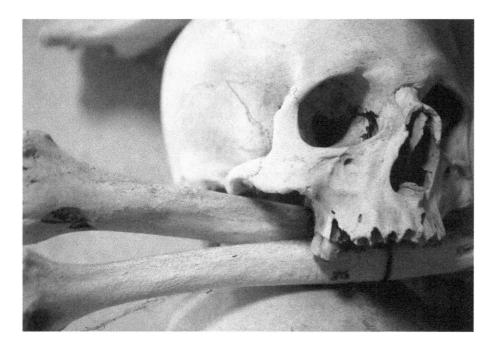

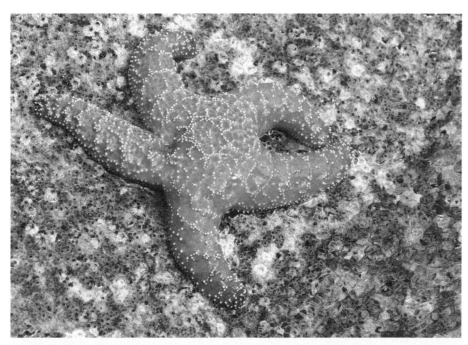

Figures 1.7/1.8

Living bone is less like desiccated, dry skeletons, and more closely resembles the adaptability of a live starfish.

evoking greater body awareness that the clients continue to notice well after their session.

Examples of techniques that feel for mobility include:

- The Carpal Scrubbing Technique (Figures 1.10 and 1.11) from Chapter 15, *The Wrist and Carpal Bones*
- The Sacroiliac Anterior/Posterior Release Technique from Chapter 13, *The Sacroiliac Joints*.

Feeling for Motility

Motility means *to be capable of motion on one's own*. Although there is cellular motility within bone tissue itself, such as the microscopic movement of osteoblasts and osteoclasts, bones are not usually thought of being able to move themselves. Bones do, however, move as a part of the body's overall motility, so the ability to feel bone movement is useful, as it is a way to perceive, assess, and affect restrictions to adaptability anywhere within the body.

When we feel for motility in bony structures, we are feeling for motion that is already happening. By contrast, when we are feeling for mobility, we are feeling for the response to movement we are inducing. Feeling for motility necessitates a quieter, even more receptive touch than mobility work, and we typically use far less pressure. The motions we feel for can include the movement of breath, or the small, adaptive movements that are always occurring at the joints. We can also feel for slower, even smaller rhythmic oscillatory motions of bones, such as the subtle motions described in craniosacral therapy. (It should be noted that very little formal research has been done on these minute cranial bone motions, and there is disagreement about their cause and even their existence. However, there is good evidence that cranial bones are capable of motion and do not fuse, as was previously thought (3).)

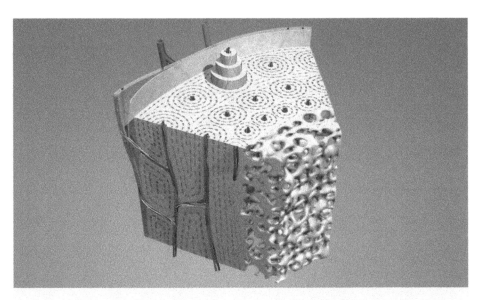

Figure 1.9

Bones are innervated and sensitive. The fibrous periosteum (outer layer) is richly innervated with mechanoreceptors; nerves (yellow) travel along with the bone's vessels, and the spongy trabeculae (innermost sections) are wound with myelinated nerve fibers.

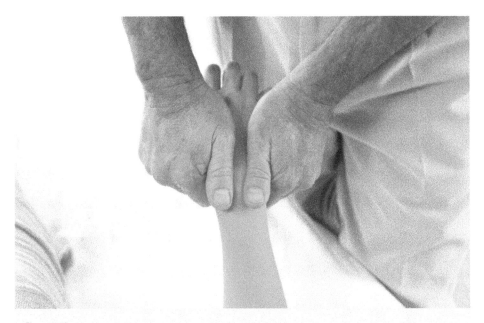

Figure 1.10

In the "Carpal Scrubbing" Technique, we feel for bony mobility, assessing each bone's anterior/posterior passive movement against its neighbors, and mobilizing those joints that move less. The bones are effective handles for working the soft tissue surrounding them, such as the carpal ligaments. This technique is described in detail in Chapter 15: The Wrist and Carpal Bones.

Tactilely "listening" for bony motion that is happening on its own is useful in the following circumstances:

1. To assess a bone or body part's degree or direction of restricted motion
2. To invite motion into an area that has been structurally released by mobility work, but that has not yet been "discovered" by the body's movement sense
3. When direct mobilization work does not yield the desired results
4. To induce a state of profound relaxation and calm, which is especially useful at the close of a session when integration and completion, rather than further release, are the goals.

Motility work is also useful when stronger mobility work might be aggravating or contraindicated (such as after acute injuries or surgery), when there is unresolved traumatic activation of the autonomic nervous system (such as with "hot" whiplash, as defined in Volume II, "Whiplash, Part 1: *Hot Whiplash*"), when touch is painful (such as in fibromyalgia, or some kinds of chronic pain), or when dealing with a taxing medical condition (such as cancer).

Motility is often subtle, and so it is sometimes challenging to detect by practitioners accustomed to more active mobilization work. However, subtle does not mean insubstantial: motility techniques can be quite tangible, profound, and effective.

One example of a motility approach is the Breath Motility Technique, in "Whiplash, Part I: *Hot Whiplash*" in Volume II.

If you are inexperienced in motility work, this technique is a great place to start, as it uses the motions of the breath, which are easily palpated.

Feeling for Connection

A third way we work with bones is by using them to feel for connection, alignment, and whole-body integration. Bones transmit force,

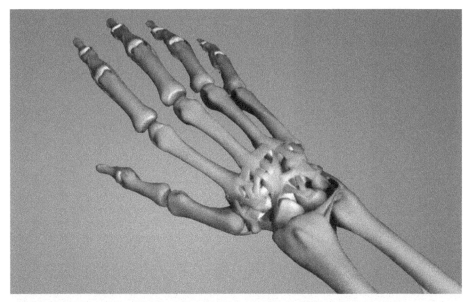

Figure 1.11

In the "Carpal Scrubbing" Technique, we feel for bony mobility, assessing each bone's anterior/posterior passive movement against its neighbors, and mobilizing those joints that move less. The bones are effective handles for working the soft tissue surrounding them, such as the carpal ligaments. This technique is described in detail in Chapter 15: The Wrist and Carpal Bones.

See video of the Breath Motility Technique at http:// advanced-trainings. com/v/ad05.html

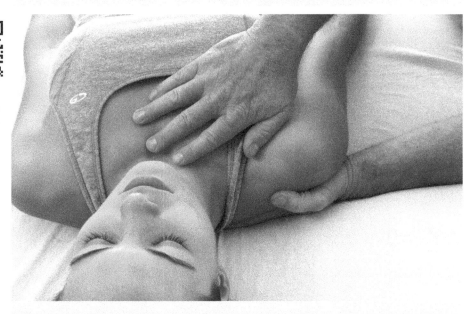

Figure 1.12

In contrast to the active touch used to feel for bony mobility, the Breath Motility Technique exemplifies a technique that uses a quieter, lighter, more receptive touch to feel for and follow movements already taking place. In this technique, the practitioner senses rib, sterna, and scapular movements accompanying the breath. When an area of less movement is found, the practitioner uses his or her touch to increase the client's awareness of that area. This technique is described in detail in Volume II.

both within their individual architecture (Figures 1.13 and 1.14), and in concert with other bones through long chains of related structures. One example of this is the transmission of the upper body's weight to the ground through the long chain of the pelvis, leg and foot bones (and conversely, the transmission of the ground's reactive force back up through these same bones in gait, jumping, and running). When bony relationships are in alignment, the compression forces of standing are borne by the skeleton, and require very little muscular effort.

We employ this principle in integrative phases of the work, such as in the Core Point of the Leg Technique (Figure 1.13), where gentle but firm static pressure is applied to a "sweet spot" just distal to the calcaneus on the sole of the foot. This sends a gentle compressive force through the limb and up through the torso. When the right spot and vector are found, the movement of this gentle pressure on the bottom of the foot will be transmitted through consecutively aligned bones, and can be seen (and felt by the client) as far up as the atlanto-occipital joint.

This principle can be applied to the upper limb as well. In the Core Point of the Arm Technique, a line of connection is found between the center of the palm and the acromion (Figure 1.14). In both the lower and upper limb variations, once the connection is found, it is held with a static touch to allow it to be registered by the client's awareness.

The purpose of this technique is to establish a proprioceptive sense of connection and integration, which is different than our previous goals of release, mobilization, listening, or following. In this way of working, the practitioner's touch serves to light up a path of aligned force transmission in the client's proprioceptive awareness, demonstrating the sensations of aligned and connected function (Figures 1.15 and 1.16). Following our artistic metaphor, you could say that the

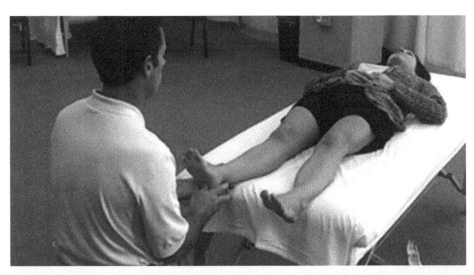

Figure 1.13
In the lower limb version of the Core Point Technique, gentle compression allows both the practitioner and the client to feel the bony connections that are part of aligned weight bearing.

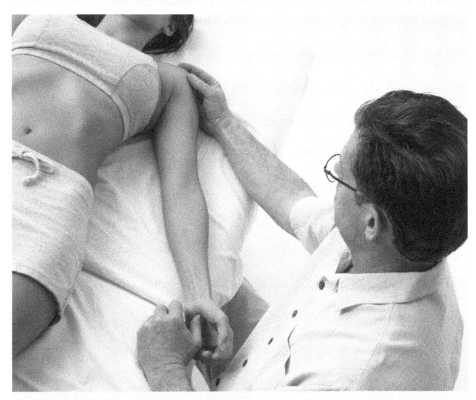

Figure 1.14
The Core Point Technique applied to the upper limb – feeling for connection between center of the palm and the acromion.

bones are the tools we use to paint on the canvas of proprioception, and we are painting a proprioceptive "image" of alignment and connection for the client's appreciation and education.

| Key points: Core Point Technique |

Indications include:
- Session closure and completion.
- Balance or proprioception issues.

Purpose
- Refine proprioception of force transmission, alignment, and inter-segmental connection through the long bones ("core") of the limbs.
- Give a sense of integration of each limb as an entirety, and of the limbs' connection to the rest of the body.

Instructions
- Use gentle but firm compressive force on the sole of the foot and palm of the hand to find a "line of transmission" through the aligned bones of the limb, so that the resulting passive movement of the body is observed (and felt by the client) through entire limb, into the torso.
- Maintain static compression of this line of transmission so as to highlight it in the client's proprioceptive awareness.

Cues
- Core Point of the Leg Technique: "How far up your body do you feel this line of connection?"
- Core Point of the Arm Technique: "How far into your torso do you feel this?"

See video of the Core Point Technique at http://advanced-trainings.com/v/ac10.html

The Core Point Technique is usually employed as a finishing move, once individual structures have been differentiated and released with mobility or motility work. It can also be adapted for the upper limb or the head.

Michelangelo's deep understanding of his medium, which was born out of his early years in the marble quarry, allowed him to make some

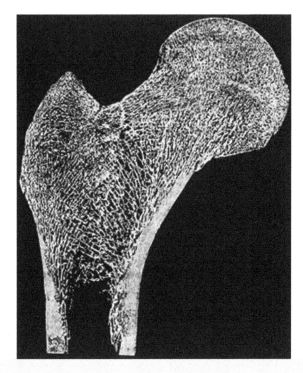

Figure 1.15

The lattice-like trabeculae inside hollow bones trace lines of compression and tension forces.

of the most compelling and enduring sculptures in Western art. Although we all have a long way to go before we begin to come close to Michelangelo's mastery, spending time in the quarry with the fundamentals of our work can help our own genius flourish, at any stage of our practice and work.

References

[1] Buehler, Markus J. (2007) Molecular nanomechanics of nascent bone: fibrillar toughening by mineralization. *Nanotechnology.* 18(29) p.2.

[2] Miller, M.R. & Kasahara, M. (1963) Observations on the innervations of human long bones. *Anat Rec.* 145 p. 13–23. doi: 10.1002/ar.1091450104.

[3] Rogers, J.S. and Witt, P.L. (1997) The controversy of cranial bone motion. *J Orthop Sports Phys Ther.* 26(2) p. 95–103.

Picture credits

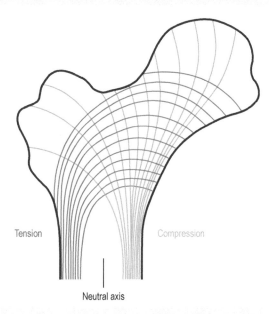

Tension   Compression

Neutral axis

Figure 1.16

Gentle pressure along the neutral axis of a limb stimulates our clients' proprioceptive sense of aligned weight transmission and connection.

Study Guide

Bone

1 As mentioned in the text, the innervated outer covering of bone is referred to as:

a trabeculae
b periosteum
c apatite
d matrix

2 According to the text, when working to increase mobility the practitioner's touch is usually:

a light
b indirect
c firm
d static

3 The text states that motility work (as distinct from mobility work) necessitates which type of touch from the practitioner?

a active
b manipulative
c firm
d receptive

4 The text suggests working with which approach when there is unresolved traumatic activation of the autonomic nervous system?

a motility
b mobility
c increasing joint range of motion
d increasing muscle tonus

5 The purpose of the Carpal Scrubbing Technique, as referred to in the text, is to increase:

a motility
b connection
c passive touch
d mobility

For Answer Keys, visit www.Advanced-Trainings.com/v1key/

What is the most abundant tissue in the body? Did you say "bone"? Good guess – after all, we have around 206 bones. Or "muscle" perhaps? It is true that we have somewhere between 600 and 800 named muscles, depending on who is counting. But even more profuse are the *fasciae* – the membranous connective tissues that surround, connect, and invest each bone and muscle, as well as every organ, vessel, and nerve (Figure 2.1). And yet, instead of having hundreds or thousands of fasciae, some say we have just one.

Fascia is famous. Growing numbers of conferences, scholarly studies, magazine articles, television specials, exercise systems, and self-help books are dedicated to the new science of fascia. Fascial theories are significantly influencing chiropractic, acupuncture, osteopathy, sports conditioning, yoga and, of course, massage and manual therapy. One sign of this is the ever-increasing number of modalities, media, manuals, and seminars focusing on fascial and myofascial approaches (including our own Advanced Myofascial Techniques series).

Fascia's fame is new. Although fascia's importance has had champions as far back as Andrew Taylor Still (1828–1917, the originator of osteopathy) and Ida P. Rolf (1898–1979, the founder of Rolfing structural integration), their emphasis on fascia was unconventional. Until relatively recently, fascia was considered a throw-away tissue – the whitish "packing material" that anatomists removed and discarded in dissections and illustrations. However, the change in our thinking about fascia has been significant. Annual numbers of peer-reviewed papers about fascia in scientific journals grew five-fold between 1970 and 2010 (1).

Systems thinking

The recent interest in fascia as a systemic, whole-body integrator is congruent with a larger-scale cultural shift in the understanding of complexity, interconnection, and whole systems. In physics, this shift in thinking can be traced back as far as Einstein, whose revolutionary Theory of Relativity supplanted Newton's mechanical, parts-based ideas of cause and effect. Gradually since that time, but especially in the last 20 years, fields as diverse as economics, environmental science, warfare, multinational trade, brain science, meteorology and climate studies, organizational psychology, business management, family therapy, nutrition, and medicine have all experienced radical revisions of their fundamental paradigms as a result of whole-system understanding. In addition, we live with far more complexity and interconnectedness than we did just 20 years ago. The emergence of the Internet is an obvious example of how a complex and widely distributed system – in some ways not unlike the interconnected fascial network of the body – has shifted our understanding of complexity. It is an understatement to say that the Internet has significantly changed how we think about our interconnections on a daily basis and, as a result, compared with 50 or even 20 years ago, we are collectively more familiar and comfortable with the idea that systems are greater than the sum of their parts; that resilience and adaptability arise from being highly interconnected; that small individual changes can have large effects in sometimes unpredictable ways; and that cause and effect are not always linear. As our way of thinking about interconnection changes, it is probably no accident that the fascia's unique properties of ubiquity and interrelatedness are at last gaining currency in orthopedic and manual therapy circles.

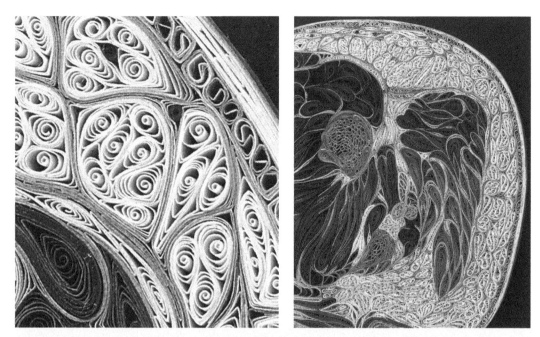

Figure 2.1

Artist Lisa Nilsson reinterprets anatomical cross-sections using rolled paper, simulating the interconnected fascial wrappings around and within muscles, bones, nerves, etc.

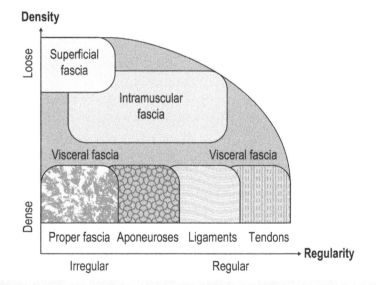

Figure 2.2

Fascia has come to refer to several types of connective tissues that vary in their density (vertical scale) and fiber regularity (horizontal scale). Not shown here are the retinaculae and joint capsules, whose properties may range between those of ligaments, aponeuroses, and proper fascia.

What is fascia?

The term *fascia* (from Latin "band") generally applies to the fibrous connective tissues covering, connecting, and investing muscles, tendons, bones, vessels, organs, and nerves. It has many subtypes, which can vary from dense to loose, and from highly regular to very irregular (Figure 2.2). Academics still debate precisely which tissues can justifiably be considered fascia (2), but researchers generally agree that all of the tissues under discussion are composed of the same basic elements (fibers, cells, and a matrix or ground substance) in varying proportions and arrangements, and that all of these tissues interconnect. Fascial researcher Robert Schleip and his collaborators offer a commonly accepted definition of fascia, saying that it is the "soft tissue components of the connective tissue system that permeates the human

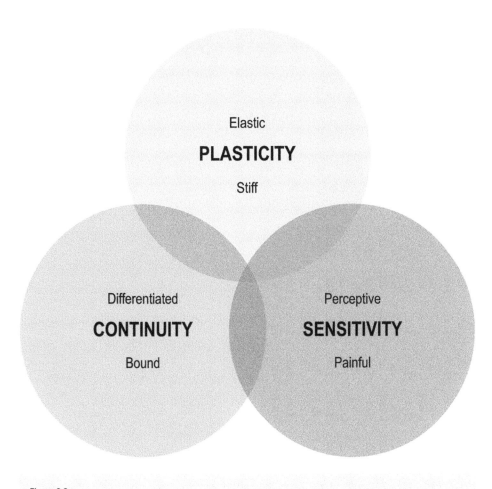

Elastic

PLASTICITY

Stiff

Differentiated

CONTINUITY

Bound

Perceptive

SENSITIVITY

Painful

Figure 2.3
Three interconnected fascial qualities relevant to hands-on work. Each quality has a beneficial and a detrimental aspect. For example, dysfunctional continuity leads to over-connection, binding, and restriction. Unhealthy plasticity takes the form of tissue that is either too dense, or too loose. And one of the downsides of fascia's sensitivity is that it can become overly sensitive to pain.

body" (3). This broad definition includes not just the enveloping membranes, but also the joint capsules, aponeuroses, ligaments, and tendons. We will use this broader interpretation in our discussion.

Myofascia

What then, is "myofascia"? Strictly speaking, myofascia refers to the fascial connective tissues related to the skeletal muscles (*myo* meaning muscle) – their internal fascial structures, external coverings, septa, and connections. Informally, myofascia is often used synonymously with fascia (though by most definitions, there are many kinds of fascia not directly related to the muscles). At Advanced-Trainings.com, we use the term "myofascial techniques" to include the active, or "myo", element of our approach. In many of our techniques, we employ active client movements in order to: a) mobilize and differentiate layers and structures that would be difficult to access passively; b) allow clients to modulate the intensity of the work; and c) reeducate neuromuscular movement patterns, as clients learn to move in new ways under the practitioner's hands.

The ups and downs of fascia

Fascia has several qualities that are particularly relevant to hands-on work. Three of these are:

I. Continuity
II. Plasticity
III. Sensitivity.

Each of these qualities could be thought of as having a beneficial and a detrimental aspect, or an upside and a downside (Figure 2.3). We will discuss each of these qualities in turn, and list the techniques that utilize each of these qualities. In the next chapter, we will then describe additional fascial techniques in greater detail.

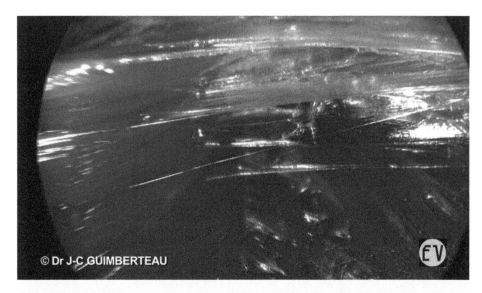

Figure 2.4

Fascial interconnections of the latissimus dorsi in a living body. About 30% of muscles' fascial connections are to other fascia, rather than to bone. This fascial continuity can be beneficial (as in force distribution), or detrimental (when unnecessary connections can bind and restrict).

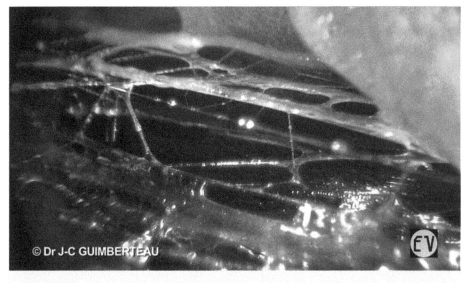

Figure 2.5

Plastic and hand surgeon Jean Claude Guimberteau's microscope shows the complex and dynamic interconnections within loose fascia of the arm.

I. Continuity

Fascia is good at connecting things together. Anatomy students are taught that fascia connects individual muscle cells to bones in an uninterrupted chain that includes the endomysium, perimysium, epimysium, tendon, and periosteum. This is true, but not quite the whole story; less well known is that about 30 percent of a muscle's fascial attachments connect to neighboring fascial structures, rather than directly to a bone (4). This fascia connects in turn to other fasciae, and so on, forming a complex three-dimensional network of multiplied interconnections (Figures 2.4 and 2.5), instead of the one-to-one linear chains usually used to describe muscular attachments. This non-linear, multidimensional fascial interconnectedness has its advantages, such as more even load distribution, tensional responsiveness, and increased overall sensitivity – similar to the idea that a fly wriggling in a well-tensioned spider's web can be sensed throughout the web's network (Figure 2.6).

In spite of being a good connector, healthy fascia is also very good at facilitating movement. It does this by being springy and elastic (see Chapter 9, *Hamstring Injuries*), and by interspersing its tough, collagenous fibers with layers of slippery proteins like proteoglycan gel, which both connects and lubricates movement between the structures that the fascia envelopes (Figure 2.5).

However, when there is strain, injury, disease, or a lack of movement, fascia responds by connecting even more, forming restrictions, scars, and adhesions. In these situations, fascia becomes overly linked with its surrounding structures, and when this happens, it binds, restricts, and pulls, much like a too-tight garment or wetsuit. Whether they are aware of it or not, clients feel this when they move, and to a trained practitioner, fascial binding can be perceived as a mobility restriction, or palpated as thicker, denser, or less-plastic regions of fascia.

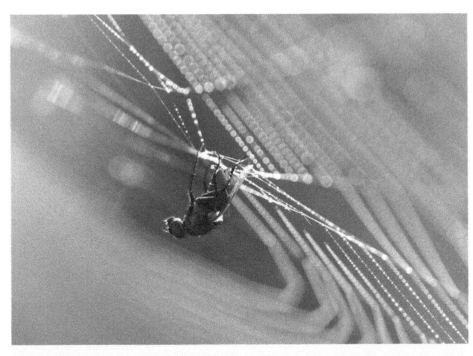

Figure 2.6

Much like a taught spider's web, the body's fascial continuity is adjusted and tuned by the muscles. This is thought to allow its sensitivity as a sensory organ to be continuously modulated. Like a fly in a web, over-connection disrupts the network's adaptability and ability to perceive.

When fascia has become overly connected, our therapeutic goal is to restore differentiation – that is, to separate fascial structures and reestablish their ability to move independently from each other. Differentiation techniques increase freedom between fascial structures through the use of active client movements to slide adjacent structures against each other, while the practitioner sensitively uses pressure or friction to gently free this movement at the fascial divisions between muscles, tendons, and other structures.

Examples of techniques for restoring fascial differentiation include:

- The Tibialis Anterior Technique from Chapter 5, "Ankle Mobility, Part II"; and
- The Hamstring Technique from Chapter 9, *Hamstring Injuries*.

The next chapter is slated to include additional techniques that help to reestablish a balance of fascial continuity and differentiation.

II. Plasticity

Practitioners feel fascia changing: with appropriate pressure and patience; tissues soften, lengthen and separate, and harder and denser areas melt away and become more pliable. Clients feel these changes too, and report tangible therapeutic effects: less pain, greater flexibility, and easier movement. "Fascial plasticity" is commonly cited as the explanation for these felt changes and, yet, the scientific explanation for what we are feeling remains under debate. Is it mechanical, neurological, or just imagined? All of these explanations have their adherents.

Thixotropy

With a PhD in biochemistry, Ida Rolf taught that the changes her deep work produced were due to a gel-to-sol melting in fascia's extracellular ground substance: in other words, the mechanical result of the practitioner's pressure. In this model, the thinning or *thixotropy* of the tissues' matrix allowed for remodeling and reorganization of the tissues and, by extension, the body in its entirety (5). Generations of structural integration practitioners – this author included – learned and taught that tissue change happened via this mechanical explanation.

Many fascial researchers (though not all) now doubt the thixotropy model, at least as a literal explanation of permanent tissue change. As tissue research has progressed since Rolf's time (she earned her biochemistry PhD in 1920), several researchers (6) have concluded that the pressure and time needed to produce tissue changes would need to be far greater than is possible in a manual therapy setting. Fascial researcher, Rolfer Robert Schleip, sums up this idea with his droll observation that during the time it has taken you to read a chapter like this one, your own bottom has been subjected to more pressure for a longer duration than most therapists ever use with their clients; yet when we stand up, most of our behinds are not flattened or deformed from our hours of daily sitting (Figure 2.1). Fascial change and plasticity clearly involves more than just mechanical pressure.

Although she continued to teach it throughout her lifetime, Rolf herself acknowledged that the thixotropy model was speculation on her part (at one point, she called her own use of the gel-to-sol analogy "nonsense teaching" and "absurd"). She also accurately predicted that the question of exactly how fascia changes would be clarified by future research (7).

While thixotropy as a literal explanation of tissue change has been called into question, other influential teachers and writers continue to use it as a conceptual model. Italian physiotherapist, Luigi Stecco, uses a combination of pressure and friction-produced heat to "maintain the fluidity of the ground substance of the deep fascia,

in such a way that the bundles of collagen fibers glide independently" (8).

Other researchers have speculated that changes in the ground substance's hydration produce the effects felt by manual therapists. Using nuclear magnetic resonance imaging, droplets of liquid water can be seen emerging on the surface of in vivo tendons during stretching (9). Since water plays an important role in fascial stiffness via the elastic interactions between protein fibers, a sponge-like wringing and refilling of the tissue's matrix is one modern alternative to the gel-sol thixotropy model.

Does fascia contract?

In the conventional view, muscles actively contract, but fascia passively resists. However, could the "release" or change in tonus felt by fascial practitioners be the relaxing of an undiscovered active contractile property of the fascia itself? Once again, we turn to Robert Schleip, who in his search for answers to this riddle, is credited with discovering actual smooth muscle-like cells within fascia, showing that fascia does actively contract after all. However, it turns out that even though the effects of these small smooth muscle cells might be within the range of what can be manually palpated, they are too weak and too slow to fully explain the tissue changes commonly observed in manual therapies (10).

So what are we feeling when we perceive fascial change under our hands? Schleip lists the aforementioned hydration changes, as well as skeletal muscle relaxation being transmitted through the fascial network, as his favored explanations for the apparent fascial change in manual therapy, adding that it could even be an imagined or ideomotor effect caused by the practitioner's subconscious expectations (11). Others are decidedly agnostic; in their chapter on fascial palpation for the book *Fascia: The Tensional Network of the Body* (the definitive reference on fascia and manual therapy), myofascial teachers Leon Chaitow and Thomas Myers (together with professors Patrick Coughlin and Thomas Findley), say of thixotropy simply that "at this time, the reported palpation experiences of manual therapists remain unexplained" (12).

Elasticity

When its plastic nature causes fascia to become stiffer or inelastic, whether due to strain, injury, scarring, disease, or lack of movement, our therapeutic goal is to restore elasticity. One technique that uses this principle is: The Rotator Cuff Technique from Chapter 18, *Frozen Shoulder, Part 2: The Rotator Cuff.*

Even if there is still disagreement about the exact mechanism involved, there is ample empirical and research-based evidence that manual therapy can increase fascial flexibility and adaptability, and that client benefits include increased mobility and less pain. After all, Ida Rolf reminded her students to not confuse their ideas about reality with reality itself by quoting scientist Alfred Korzybski's dictum that "The map is not the territory." Whichever model or map we use to explain the tissue effects of our work, and whether we think of that model as scientific fact or an inspirational metaphor, practitioners continue to feel the tissue melting under our hands. And, most importantly, our clients continue to experience less pain, easier movement, and more flexibility.

III. Sensitivity

If you were to draw your own body, not as you see it from the outside, but as you feel it from the inside, what would it look like? You might have to close your eyes to imagine this, but ask yourself – what is the overall "image" of your body sensations, from the inside-out? Take a moment to do this now.

Once you have a sense of this, the next question is, "What is it that you are sensing your body *with*?" When we look at ourselves in the mirror, we use our eyes; when we "look" at ourselves from the inside, what sense-organ are we using? There is good evidence that, more than any other single source, we feel our body using the many mechanoreceptors and nerve endings in our fascia (13). The fasciae have so many sensory receptors that (depending on how you count them) their total number could equal or surpass that of the retina of the eye, which is usually considered the richest human sensory organ (14).

Of course, other tissues contribute to our felt body sense: the bones have sensation (much of it from its fascial wrapping, or periosteum), as do joint capsules (though some classification systems consider joint capsule tissue to be a type of fascia). The organs have sensation, although they are not particularly sensitive compared to other tissues (on the other hand, the visceral fasciae, which cover each organ, are especially rich in sensory free nerve endings). Muscle tissue itself is also sensitive, though once again, the fascial network that invests and surrounds every muscle, muscle cell, and fiber, has about six times as many sensory nerve receptors as muscle tissue itself (15).

Skin is very sensitive, especially to exteroception (perceiving the outside world through the sense of touch), but the perception of sensation from within the body begins just under the skin's dermis. The tissues in this zone, which include the superficial and deeper fascial membranes and their adjacent spaces (Figure 2.5), are exceptionally dense with free nerve endings and mechanoreceptors (Figure 2.5 and 2.7) (16). These sense pressure, stretching, shearing, vibration, and so on, and help us perceive, control, and coordinate our movements, while also allowing us to shape the felt sense of our physical selves.

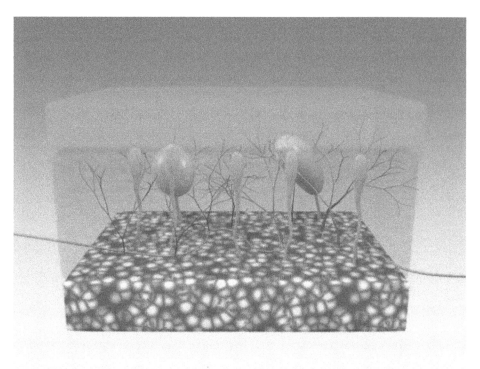

Figure 2.7

Fascial layers are often richly embedded with free nerve endings and other mechanoreceptors, such as the Pacinian corpuscles (pictured here in the superficial fascia and hypodermis), as well as the Ruffini endings in deeper fascia.

Fascia's sensitivity means that it is also sensitive to pain. While a benefit of pain is that it can help us avoid further injury, fascial sensitivity may play a role in chronic pain that persists longer than is biologically useful. Sometimes, fascial pain is related to direct trauma, because it is often more sensitive than the structures it envelopes; the pain from tears or strains is often felt most acutely in the fascia. This is also seen in the link between some kinds of low back pain and the thoracolumbar fascia (17). Other times, fascia seems to play a role in generating or sustaining pain, such as with trigger points or myofascial pain syndrome (MPS). Though MPS is complex and not fully understood, manual therapies have been observed to help (18). Several writers (19) speculate that fascial stiffness plays a role in MPS and other chronic pain by stimulating embedded nociceptors. Fascial anatomist Antonio Stecco cites evidence for this hypothesis from ultrasound experiments where neck pain was proportional to fascial thickness which, in turn, responded to fascial manipulation (20).

Fascia's sensitivity has implications beyond pain and proprioception. Schleip observes that patients under a general anesthetic have greater movement in many joints than they do while awake (21), suggesting that sensitivity (via the nervous system) plays a significant role in movement restrictions that might otherwise be explained as mechanical or structural stiffness.

In our manual therapy approach, we use fascia's sensitivity in a variety of ways:

- We use fascial proprioceptors to alter the resting tone of muscles and the tension of their associated connective tissues. Many of our techniques use static pressure on musculotendinous and periosteal attachments. Combining this pressure with active client movement stimulates Golgi tendon organs and other mechanoreceptors, which modify the motor tonus of associated muscles (22). One technique that employs this principle is the Push Broom "A" Technique (from Chapter 10, *Hip Mobility*).

- Skin-to-skin touch can calm the autonomic nervous system's (ANS) sympathetic fight or flight arousal, and it has profound impacts on psychological well-being (23). Although deep work that is overly painful has been shown to have an opposite, stress-like effect on ANS sympathetic activation, skilled work with deep fascia receptors (such as the Ruffini corpuscles, which respond to deep, slow touch) can calm fight-or-flight responses (24). The Cervical Translation Technique (slated for inclusion in Volume II) uses deep fascial sensation to, among other goals, calm sympathetic activation.

- One of the primary goals of our work, no matter what technique is used, is to help clients refine the perceptive capability of their felt body sense (proprioception, interoception, exteroception, and so on). The benefits of increased body awareness are profound and wide reaching, ranging from more sustainable in-the-moment choices about posture and comfort, to better coordination (25), and increased overall well-being (26). We accomplish this perceptive refinement by asking clients to attend to the sensations of the work itself, to report on their sensory experience, and by other means. This way of working can inform any technique, but the Breath Motility Technique (slated for inclusion in Volume II) is an example of a technique that focuses primarily on the client's proprioception.

Areas of overlap

This chapter has introduced a few ways that fascial understanding informs our Advanced Myofascial Techniques approach. We have not attempted to catalog more than a small amount of the rapidly expanding knowledge about fascia, nor have we tried to describe other

systems' ways of working with this endlessly interesting tissue. Each of the myriad fascial, myofascial, and connective tissue approaches has its own paradigm, priorities, goals, and benefits, though the ideas we have described here are often compatible and complimentary with those of other systems.

We have described plasticity, continuity, and sensitivity as separate phenomena but, in reality, there are large areas of overlap between these three fascial qualities. For instance, it is likely that fascia's plasticity is intimately linked to its sensitivity. Moreover, fascia's sensitivity as a sense organ can be augmented (or hindered) by its web-like continuity. Finally, fascia's degree of continuity (how connected or separate it is) is directly related to its textural plasticity and elasticity. Even though describing them separately here helps us better understand and appreciate all of fascia's remarkable qualities, in practice we work with all three of these qualities simultaneously in our hands-on work – much in the same way that the fascia itself is an undivided whole.

References

[1] Schleip, R. et al. (2012) *Fascia, The Tensional Network of the Human Body*. Elsevier, p. xvi.

[2] Langevin, H.M. and Huijing, P.A. (2009) Communicating About Fascia: History, Pitfalls, and Recommendations. *Int J Ther Massage Bodywork*. 2(4). p. 3–8.

[3] 1. Schleip, R. et al. (2012) *Fascia, The Tensional Network of the Human Body*. Elsevier.

[4] Huijing, P.A. (1999) Muscular force transmission: a unified, dual or multiple system? A review and some explorative experimental results. *Arch Physiol Biochem*. 107. p. 292–311.

[5] Rolf, I. (1977) *Rolfing – the integration of the human studies*. New York: Harper and Row.

[6] Currier, D. and Nelson, R. (1992) Dynamics of human biologic tissues. FA Davis Company, Philadelphia. And, Chaudhry, H., Findley, T., Huang, C., et al. (2011) Three dimensional mathematical models for deformation of human fascia. *J. Amer. Ost. Assoc*. 108. p. 379–390.

[7] Transcript of Ida Rolf's lectures, Tape A5 (1970), Side 1, available to members on www.rolfguild.org, as cited by Paul Ingraham, http://saveyourself.ca/articles/does-fascia-matter.php#ref10 [accessed Feb 2014].

[8] Stecco, L. (2004) Fascial manipulation for musculoskeletal pain. *Piccin Nuova Libreria*. 19.

[9] Helmer, K.G., Nair, G. and Cannella, M. (2006) Water movement in tendon in response to a repeated static tensile load using one-dimensional magnetic resonance imaging. *Biomech. Eng.* 128(5). p. 733–741.

[10] Schleip, R., Kingler, W. and Lehmann- Horn, F. (2007) Fascia is able to contract in a smooth muscle-like manner and thereby influence musculoskeletal mechanics. In: Findley, T.W., Schleip, R. (Eds.), *Fascia Research Basic Science and Implications for Conventional and Complementary Health Care*. Munich: Urban and Fischer, p. 76–77.

[11] Schleip, R. (2012). Fascial Research Group FAQ. http://www.fasciare-search.de/faq#Q5. [Accessed Feb. 2014]

[12] Chaitow, L., Coughlin, P., Findley, T.W. and Myers, T. (2012) "Fascial palpation." Schleip, R. et al. *Fascia, The Tensional Network of the Human Body*. Elsevier, p. 271.

[13] Schleip, R. (2003) Fascial plasticity – a new neurobiological explanation. Part 1. *J Bodyw Mov Ther*. 7(1). p. 11–19.

[14] Mitchell, J.H. and Schmidt, R.F. (1977) Cardiovascular reflex control by afferent fibers from skeletal muscle receptors. In: Shepherd, J.T. et al., (Eds.), *Handbook of physiology, Section 2, Vol. III, Part 2*. p. 623–658.

[15] Van der Wal, J. (2009) The architecture of the connective tissue in the musculoskeletal system: An often over-looked functional parameter as to proprioception in the locomotor apparatus. In: Huijing, P.A. et al., (Eds.), *Fascia research II: Basic science and implications for conventional and complementary health care*. Elsevier GmbH, Munich, Germany.

[16] Stecco C., Porzionato, A., Lancerotto L. et al. (2008) Histological study of the deep fasciae of the limbs. *J Bodyw Mov Ther*. 12(3). p. 225–230.

[17] Barker, P.J. and Briggs, C.A. (2007) Anatomy and biomechanics of the lumbar fasciae: implications for lumbopelvic control and clinical practice. In: Vleeming, A., et al. *Movement, stability and lumbopelvic pain*. Edinburgh: Elsevier, p. 64–73.

[18] Lee, N.G. and You, J.H. (2007) Effects of trigger point pressure release on pain modulation and associated movement impairments in a patient with severe acute myofascial pain syndrome: A case report. *The Pain Clinic* 19(2) p. 83–87.

[19] LeMoon, K. (2008) Clinical Reasoning in Massage Therapy. *International Journal of Therapeutic Bodywork and Massage 1 (1)*. (http://www.ijtmb.org/index.php/ijtmb/article/view/2/20).

[20] Stecco, A., Meneghini, A., Stern, R., Stecco, C. and Imamura, M. (2013) Ultrasonography in myofascial neck pain: randomized clinical trial for diagnosis and follow-up. *Surg Radiol Anat*. Aug 23.

[21] Schleip, R. et al. (2012) *Fascia, The Tensional Network of the Human Body*. Elsevier, p. 78.

[22] Cottingham, J.T. (1985) *Healing through touch – A history and review of the physiological evidence*. Boulder, Colorado: Rolf Institute Publications.

[23] Montague, A. (1971) *Touch: the human significance of the skin*. New York: Harper & Row.

[24] Schleip, R. (2003) Fascial plasticity – a new neurobiological explanation. Part 1. *J Bodyw Mov Ther*. 7(1). p. 11–19.

[25] Langevin, H.M. (2006) Connective tissue: a body-wide signaling network? *Med. Hypotheses*. 66. p. 1074–1077.

[26] Seppälä, E. (2012) Decoding the Body Watcher. *Scientific American*. Apr 3.

Recommended reading

Schleip, R., Findley, T., Chaitow, L. and Huijing, P. (2012) *Fascia, the Tensional Network of the Human Body*. Elsevier.

Picture credits

Figure 2.1 courtesy Lisa Nilsson www.lisanilssonart.com, used by permission. Photographer: John Polak.

Figure 2.2 courtesy Robert Schleip, www.fascialnet.com, used by permission.

Figure 2.3 courtesy Advanced-Trainings.com, used by permission.

Figures 2.4 and 2.5 courtesy Jean Claude Guimberteau, used by permission.

Figures 2.6 courtesy Michal Boubin/Thinkstock, used by permission.

Figure 2.7 courtesy Hank Grebe, www.mediaspin.com, used by permission.

Study Guide

Fascia, Part 1: Understanding Fascial Change

1 When fascia has become overly connected to neighboring structures, the text states that the practitioner's aim is to:

a lessen pain
b restore differentiation
c increase flexibility
d lengthen tissue

2 The writing cites evidence that more than any other single source, we feel our own bodies via:

a our bones
b our skin
c our fascia
d our muscles

3 The text cites ultrasound evidence that correlates the severity of neck pain to:

a the number of cervical mechanoceptors
b the amount of cervical muscular tension
c the thickness of the cervical fascia
d the types of fascia present

4 To change muscle tonus via the Golgi tendon organs, this approach works on musculotendinous attachments using static pressure, in combination with what?

a passive client movement
b active client movement
c passive stretching
d a slight vibratory or pulsing motion

5 According to the text, what does fascial researcher Robert Schleip list as his favored explanation for the apparent fascial changes brought about by manual therapy?

a neurological changes triggered by Paccinian corpuscles
b thixotropic melting of the ground substance under pressure
c hydration changes and skeletal muscle relaxation
d Schleip argues that what is in fashion changes, but fascia does not

For Answer Keys, visit www.Advanced-Trainings.com/v1key/

Fascial qualities

Our last chapter "Understanding fascial change" described fascia and its qualities in detail. As a brief review, fascia can vary from dense to loose, and from very regular fiber organization (such as in the tendons or ligaments) to irregular (for example, superficial fascia (Figure 3.1) or scar tissue). These many varieties of fascia share

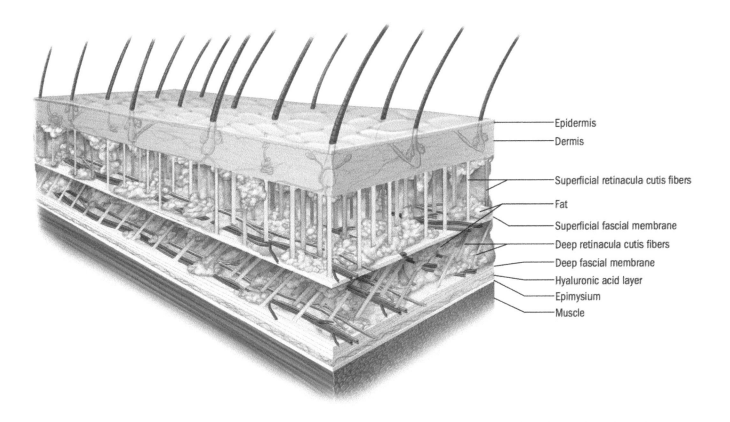

Epidermis
Dermis
Superficial retinacula cutis fibers
Fat
Superficial fascial membrane
Deep retinacula cutis fibers
Deep fascial membrane
Hyaluronic acid layer
Epimysium
Muscle

Figure 3.1

Cross-section of layers from skin to musculature, showing the fascial membranes interspersed with cells, fluids, nerves, and vessels. Note the thin layer of hyaluronic acid just under the deep fascial membrane, which allows the musculature to move freely beneath the outer layers.

several common qualities, which can change depending on the tissues' degree of health. Fascia can be stiff, bound, and painful when it has been distressed (through injury or disease), neglected (through lack of movement), or overused (by activity, posture, or habit). Skilled hands-on work can change each of these problematic qualities, thus helping the body's fascia to regain differentiation, elasticity, and refined perception. This chapter will describe two hands-on techniques that do just that.

Forearm Flexor Technique

Although there are many techniques we could use to illustrate the principles of fascial work, the Forearm Flexor Technique brings together many pieces of the fascial puzzle. The forearm is also a place where people who work with their hands (such as manual therapists) often lose differentiation, elasticity, and proprioceptive refinement, which are the three essential qualities of fascial health.

Preparation

Prepare for this technique by palpating the layers of fascia surrounding the anterior, or palm side, of the arm. Using your fingertips or pads, feel the outermost layers of tissue over the wrist and finger flexors of your client's lower arm. Do not use oil or lubricant, as you will actually be using the friction between layers to perceive and mobilize any adhesions or restrictions you may find.

At first, move just the surface layers of the lower arm, feeling how you can slide the skin on the muscles underneath. If you slow down and feel for more detail, you will be able to discern that there are multiple layers of wrappings – some clearly distinguishable, and others blending with adjacent layers. Gently stretch and move

See video of the Forearm Flexor Technique at http://advanced-trainings.com/v/aa07.html

these layers, and you will find that they slide or stretch to different degrees and in different directions.

The superficial fascia (or subcutaneous layer) lies just under the skin. Some sources reserve the term "superficial fascia" solely for the fibrous membrane between the dermis and the deeper fascia surrounding the muscles; others define the superficial fascia as including all of the looser tissue layers adjacent to this membrane. Whichever definition we use, it is here that we find the retinacula cutis fibers – the numerous and minute small skin ligaments that are arranged above and below a fibrous membrane (Figure 3.1). These tiny, column-like skin ligaments suspend this fascial membrane between the dermis above and the deeper fascia below. The varying angles of the retinacula cutis are responsible for the palpable "grain" of the superficial layers – the way in which these layers slide more easily in some directions than in others. The spaces between the retinacula cutis fibers are filled with fatty tissue, nerves and nerve endings, vasculature, and interstitial tissue fluids, giving these outer layers their looser or softer feel.

Just below these superficial layers, you can feel the deeper antebrachial fascia (Figures 3.4 and 3.9) (2). This glove-like layer is part of the deep fascia – the tough membranes that surround the entire body just under the superficial fascia, but that lie over the fascia of the muscles themselves. The deep fascia is called aponeuroses in some places, and where it dives deeper between muscles, it is referred to as the investing fascia or intermuscular septa. These contiguous structures tend to be denser and more resilient than the freer superficial layers. They are usually composed of several sub-layers of collagen fibers. Some of these fibers are arranged parallel to the muscle fibers underneath, and others are organized at oblique angles, like the layers

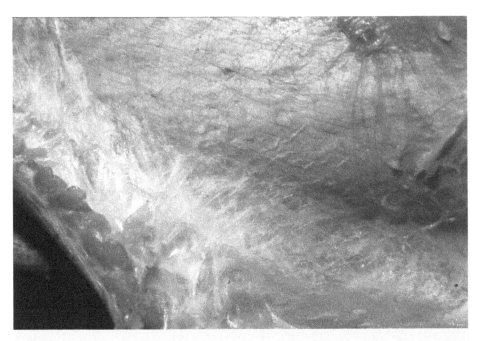

Figure 3.2
The varying fiber direction in deep fascia.

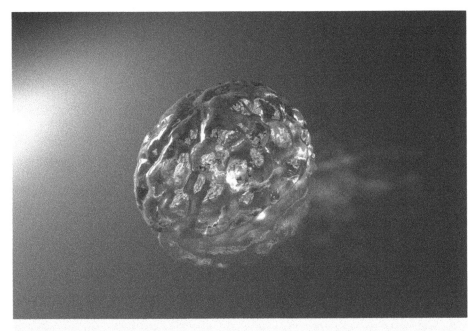

Figure 3.3
Hyaluronic acid, one of the slippery fluids that lubricates and nourishes the fascial layers and allows the musculature to move freely beneath the outer layers.

in plywood, in order to resist differing lines of force (Figure 3.2). Between the deep fascia and the fascial wrappings of the individual muscles below them (the epimysia) is a thin layer of slippery hyaluronic acid (Figure 3.3), which allows the large amount of gliding necessary for free muscular movement.

Key points: Forearm Flexor Technique

Indications include:
- Movement restrictions, pain, or paresthesia in the forearm, wrist, or hand (including neurovascular compression symptoms).

Purpose
- Increase differentiation and elasticity of fascia layers and compartments.

Instructions
- Use fingertips, soft fist, or forearm, in combination with client's active movement, to:
  1. Palpate and mobilize outer layers of forearm.
  2. Increase differentiation between forearm flexors.

Movements
- Finger flexion (all together, and individually). "Make a fist."
- Wrist flexion.

Layers Exercise

As a touch experiment, see if you can distinguish between the three different levels:

1. Skin: first, simply glide on the surface of the skin (as you would do with oil or lubricant).
2. Superficial fascia: next, barely under the surface, move only the outermost tissues as you feel for the slight sponginess, looseness, and "grain" within the superficial layers (which themselves are composed of multiple sub-layers).

27

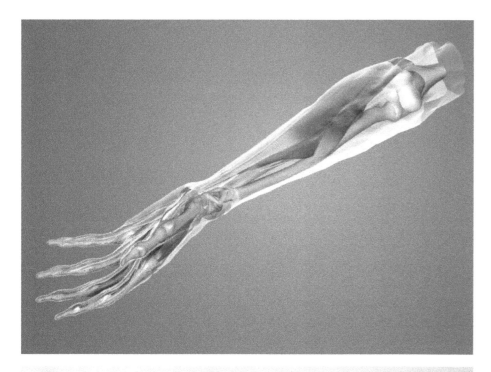

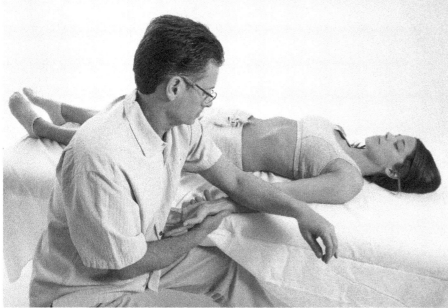

Figures 3.4/3.5

The Forearm Flexor Technique begins with the outermost layers of most arm fascia. Use the forearm tool to palpate the layers, before going deeper to gently feel between the fascial compartments of the arm.

3. Deep fascia: slightly deeper (but still not into the belly of the muscles), feel the tougher membrane that glides easily on the muscles underneath. This is the deep fascia sliding on its hyaluronic acid layer (Figure 3.1).

An analogy might be helpful: imagine a sheet on a massage table. The first level of movement would be to feel the texture of the sheet's surface; the second, the stretch and weave of the sheet fabric itself; and the third, the way the sheet slides on the table underneath.

Differentiating layers

Once you can clearly distinguish these layers from one another, switch from using your fingertips to using your forearm (Figures 3.5 and 3.6). Use the broad, flat surface of your ulna, just distal to the elbow. Avoid using the point of the elbow itself (the olecranon process) at this point. The forearm is a powerful tool, so focus mainly on perception rather than manipulation. Take some time to explore the outer layers again (Figure 3.4). Compare the lower arm's palm side, where the skin is thin and the layers are usually clearly palpable, with the thicker layers on the forearm's dorsum (back-of-the-hand side). Make sure that you are still feeling just the wrappings of the arm and that you are not yet working into the muscles themselves. This can be a challenge, especially if you are used to massaging muscles rather than differentiating fascia. Feel for places where the outer layers are thicker, or where they do not seem to slide against one another. Try moving in a proximal direction (as shown in Figures 3.5 and 3.6), as well as distally, medially, and laterally, in order to feel the differing fiber direction at various depths. When you find such places, gently move them in the more difficult direction (a direct release, as opposed to moving in the easier direction, which would invite an indirect release), and wait for a change.

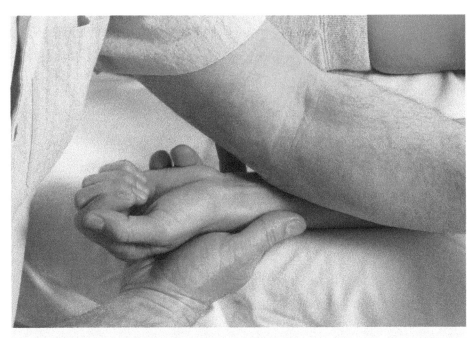

Figure 3.6

Actively closing and opening the hand in the Forearm Flexor Technique will further differentiate layers and compartments.

In addition to increasing your skill at palpating specific tissue layers, this slow, specific mobilization of the arm's outer wrappings has therapeutic effects. Moving layer on layer helps accomplish our fascial goal of differentiation, as these layers will become freer and more slippery the longer you work them. You will notice that the slower you move, the more fluid the tissue feels; go slow enough, and tissue restrictions seem to melt away on their own, which brings in greater elasticity (our second facial goal). As the outer fascial layers are so rich with free nerve endings and other mechanoreceptors, we are also stimulating facial sensitivity and perception (our third goal).

Differentiating compartments

Once you have thoroughly explored the outer fascial layers that wrap the lower arm, sink a bit deeper. Keep the same sensitivity to layering and fiber direction. Rather than just "mashing" the muscles until they are softer everywhere, use the tip of your forearm to gently feel down in between the muscles, looking for the spaces between the various muscular compartments and bundles (Figure 3.8). The consistency and density of the wrappings, septa, and intramuscular fascia that define these bundles can vary, but they are often thicker, firmer, and more adhered into a single mass in people who use their arms or hands for repeated motions, like gripping, typing, and so on. As with the outer wrappings, our aim is to encourage both elasticity and differentiation, so feel for stiffer areas of tissue and for any places where bundles or layers do not seem to slide against one another. Your pressure is firm and specific, but never so much that your client has to tense or withdraw in any way. When you find a motion-restricted area, wait patiently with static pressure, or glide just a bit, at a super-slow pace, until you feel a softening or easing response in the tissue.

To get even better differentiation between the arm flexors, ask your client to slowly flex and extend

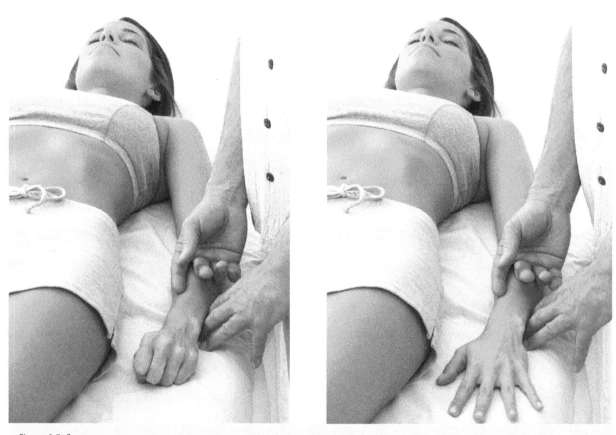

Figures 3.7a/b

In the Forearm Extensor Technique, use the knuckles of your soft fist to differentiate the outer fascial layers of the arm. Ask for active finger and wrist movements to help differentiate the deeper fascial compartments between the muscles of the forearm.

his or her wrist, or open and close his or her hand (Figure 3.6). With your own forearm, continue to search for the furrows and separation between muscle bundles. Sensitively and slowly, you can use the tip of your elbow a bit more now to feel between the forearm's muscular compartments. Ask the client to participate by making individual finger motions, as if playing the piano or typing. This will allow you to more accurately feel the individual flexors, and to sink between them as your client moves. Use much gentler pressure over the wrist, of course, and do not use so much pressure or speed that you cause pain. You can get all the therapeutic effects we have discussed by being patient and focused, rather than heavy

and fast. Continue this work throughout the entire flexor surface of the lower arm.

Forearm Extensor Technique

Once you have differentiated the tissue layers and muscle bundles on the anterior (palm) side of the lower arm, repeat the process on the posterior side. The majority of muscles in this region relate to finger and wrist extension, though you will also find thumb and elbow muscles here.

Given that the posterior side of the arm is less fleshy and more sensitive than the anterior side, we will use a different tool: the soft fist. Keeping your fingers open and your wrist straight (Figures 3.7a and

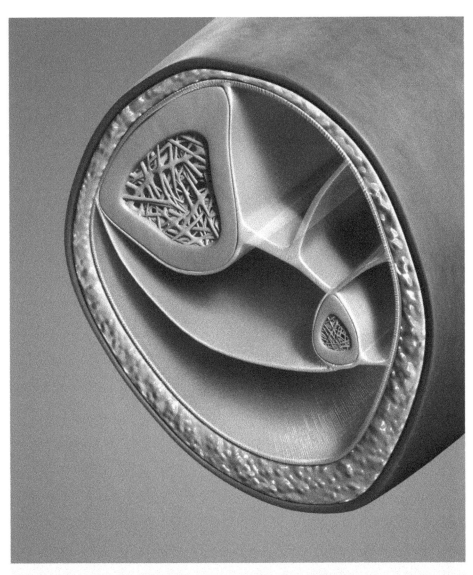

Figure 3.8

The fascial compartments of the lower leg, where the compartmental architecture is similar to the lower arm.
Illustration courtesy of fascialnet.com.

37.b) will allow you to work sensitively and deeply with very little effort. The skin of the knuckles is hard and smooth enough to allow for good control while gliding layer over layer when working the antebrachial fascia (Figures 3.4 and 3.9). Once you have worked the superficial layers, the shape of your knuckles allows you to gently sink between the extensor compartments in the forearm (similar to those pictured in Figure 3.8) in order to separate and differentiate their structure and function.

Again, ask for slow, steady wrist and finger movement, in all directions. As before, invite your client to use these active movements to further differentiate between the fascial structures on the extensor side. Examples of ways to cue this exploration might be: "Let your fingers flex and extend, one at a time, as if playing a scale on the piano," or "Pretend you're typing. Find the finger movements that are harder than others, and play with those" (Figure 3.7a/b).

In addition to the mechanical effects of increased differentiation and elasticity, the combination of slow active movement and pressure floods your

Key points: Forearm Extensor Technique

Indications include:
- Movement restrictions or pain in the forearm, wrist, or hand.

Purpose
- Increase differentiation and elasticity of fascia layers and compartments.

Instructions
- Use fingertips, soft fist, or forearm, in combination with client's active movement, to:
  1. Palpate and mobilize outer layers of forearm.
  2. Increase differentiation between forearm extensors.

Movements
a. Finger extension (all and individually). Cues: "Flatten your hand onto the table." "Lift one finger at a time."
b. Wrist extension.

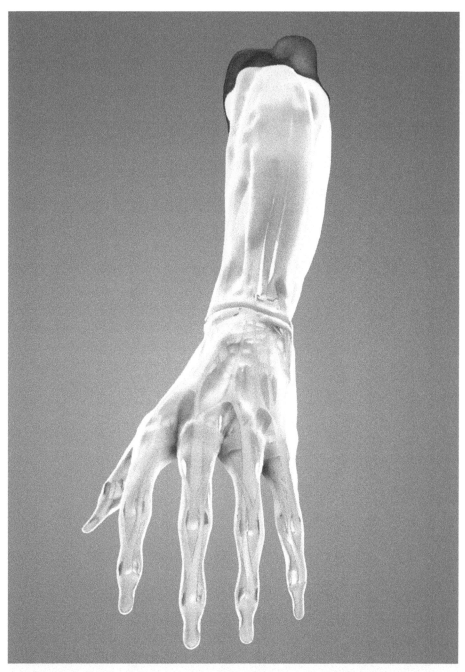

Figure 3.9

Extensor compartments in the forearm.

client's brain with novel sensation related to proprioception and movement control. Imagine that you are turning up the volume on the signals your client uses for proprioceptive coordination. When you find a movement limitation, for example, one finger extending less than the others, you can use this combination of focused pressure and proprioceptive refinement to evoke new movement possibilities. The changes in range of motion and refined control are often dramatic, and because they involve neuromuscular learning as well as tissue change, these changes tend to last over time.

Antebrachial Fascia Technique

Up to this point in our discussion on fascial tools and techniques, we have mostly worked to distinguish and differentiate between fascial layers in areas where they are adhered or conjoined. Thus far, our techniques have been directed at feeling and releasing specific restrictions. As a counterpoint to this local specificity, we will take a more global approach in our final example. This broadening of our focus is appropriate for the closing, integration phases of our work, as it leaves the client with an enhanced sense of the body as a connected, interrelated whole.

As mentioned, the antebrachial fascia is much like a gauntlet or full-length glove of deep fascia that surrounds the entire lower arm (Figures 3.4 and 3.9). This sheath of dense, fibrous tissue is continuous with the deep fascia layer that surrounds the entire body. Over the wrist, its thickenings are known as the extensor and flexor retinacula, which play important roles in hand and carpal function (see Chapter 15, The Wrist and Carpal Bones). The underside of the antebrachial fascia gives off many intermuscular septa, which are the structures we worked to differentiate in the previous techniques.

We will introduce an additional fascial tool here: the fingertips. With curled (slightly flexed) fingers, grip the tough layer of the antebrachial fascia, both anteriorly and posteriorly. Feel for a three-dimensional sense of this surrounding layer's continuity around the arm. Without sliding on the surface of the skin, move the deep fascial membrane on its layer of slick hyaluronic acid, which separates it from the muscular fascia just underneath (Figure 3.1). As with the Layers exercise, feel for adhesions and places of restricted mobility. Less mobility is normal where the antebrachial fascia attaches the ulna, both along its entire posterior edge and at the olecranon. However, since our focus is broader and more global, keep the entire layer's continuity in your awareness, rather than focusing solely on the local restrictions.

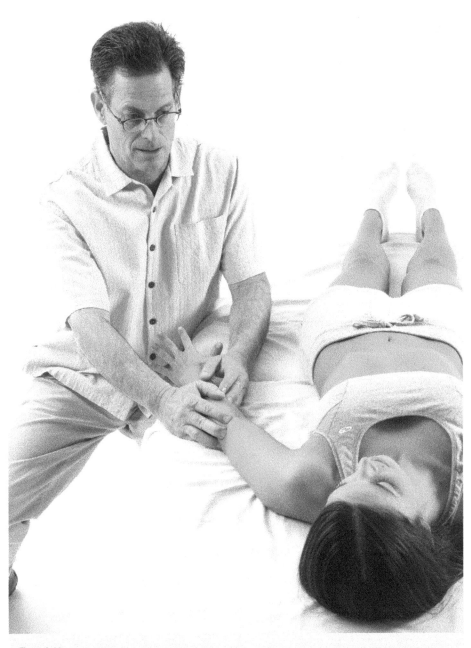

Figure 3.10

In the Antebrachial Fascia Technique, use your fingertips to continue the layer differentiation that you began in the earlier techniques, and to give a sense of overall continuity and connection. Cue your client to gently lengthen his or her arm, as if slowly extending it into a sleeve.

Key points: Antebrachial Fascia Technique

Indications include:

- Unrefined, all-or-nothing upper limb movement initiation.
- Upper limb session closure; integration.

Purpose

- Differentiation of the antebrachial fascia from deeper epimysial layers.
- Neuromuscular reeducation of shoulder movement initiation patterns.

Instructions

1. Use fingertips to anchor antebrachial fascia on anterior and posterior sides of arm. Use slight proximal pressure, without gliding or slipping.
2. Feel for this layer's ability to glide on the fascial layers below it when client actively lengthens the arm.

Cues

- "Let your arm get longer."
- "Allow your hand to initiate the motion, so that it moves before your shoulder contracts."
- "Relax your shoulders onto the table."

Apply a slight proximal traction to this layer, using just a bit of your fingernail to anchor your grip. At the same time, ask your client to gently extend (lengthen) his or her arm, as if reaching into a glove or sleeve (Figure 3.10). This provides some counter-force against your distal traction.

Make sure your client's shoulder stays relaxed; cue your client to begin the motion at the hand, rather than at the shoulder. Small movements are often more effective than larger ones. This subtle, distally initiated movement will allow for a sense of lengthening and ease throughout the entire upper limb, instead of requiring the type of muscular effort that comes from initiating gross movement at the shoulder.

Although the counter-pressure and resistance you and your client provide each other does help differentiate the antebrachial fascia from its surrounding layers, we also have the goal of increasing proprioceptive refinement. In this case, we are educating our client about how to begin movement in the upper limb without unnecessary shoulder girdle involvement.

Wrap-up

Although there are many tools for working with fascia, I have described just three examples here: the forearm, the soft fist, and the fingertips. As a set, these three tools will provide you with effective ways to invite greater fascial differentiation and elasticity almost anywhere in the body. The forearm is well suited for large areas, such as the fascia over the spinal erectors or the iliotibial tract. The soft fist is useful for detailed work, such as the superficial fasciae of the neck, the plantar fascia, and so on. Finally, the fingertips allow you to move one layer on another with unparalleled effectiveness, which is useful when working with the deep fascia anywhere in the body, particularly with the retinacula around the wrists and ankles.

The other important "tool" we have used for working with fascia is your client's active movement. By asking your client to feel into the work and move in a way that facilitates differentiation and elasticity, we leverage fascia's perceptive qualities in the service of lasting change.

References

[1] Schleip, R. et al. (2012) Fascia, *The Tensional Network of the Human Body*. Elsevier. p. xvi.

[2] Stecco, C. et al. (2009) The Palmaris longus muscle and its relations with the antebrachial fascia and the palmar aponeurosis. *Clin Anat.* Mar 22 (2). p. 221–229.

Picture credits

3.1 courtesy Joe Muscolino. Originally published in the *Massage Therapy Journal,* Body Mechanics column, Spring 2012. Used with permission.
Figure 3.2 courtesy Ron Thompson. Used with permission.
Figure 3.3 Thinkstock.
Figures 3.4 and 3.10 courtesy Primal Pictures. Used with permission.
Figures 3.5, 3.6, 3.7a/b, and 3.10 courtesy Advanced-Trainings.com.
Figure 3.8 courtesy Robert Schleip, © www.fascialnet.com. Used with permission.

Study Guide

Fascia, Part 2: Fascial Tools and Techniques

1 **Why does the author recommend not using lubrication for the techniques in this chapter?**

a to better distinguish the myofascial approach from massage therapy
b to stimulate rather than relax the nervous system
c to better perceive and mobilize fascial restrictions or adhesions
d the rationale for not using oil is not given

2 **According to the text, what creates the "grain" or the way in which the superficial layers of fascia slide easier in some directions than others?**

a the thixotropic effect
b the nervous system
c the hyaluronic acid layer
d the retinacula cutis fibers

3 **As described in the chapter, which layer is suspended between the superficial and deep retinacula cutis layers?**

a the superficial fascial membrane
b the antebrachial fascia
c the epimysium
d the hyaluronic acid layer

4 **When the practitioner finds a motion-restricted area while differentiating fascial compartments, the text recommends:**

a waiting patiently with static pressure
b using more pressure
c using less pressure
d working deeper

5 **In the Forearm Flexor Technique, what are the client's active movements?**

a flex and extend the elbow
b pronate and supinate the forearm
c abduct and adduct the wrist
d flex and extend the wrist

For Answer Keys, visit www.Advanced-Trainings.com/v1key/

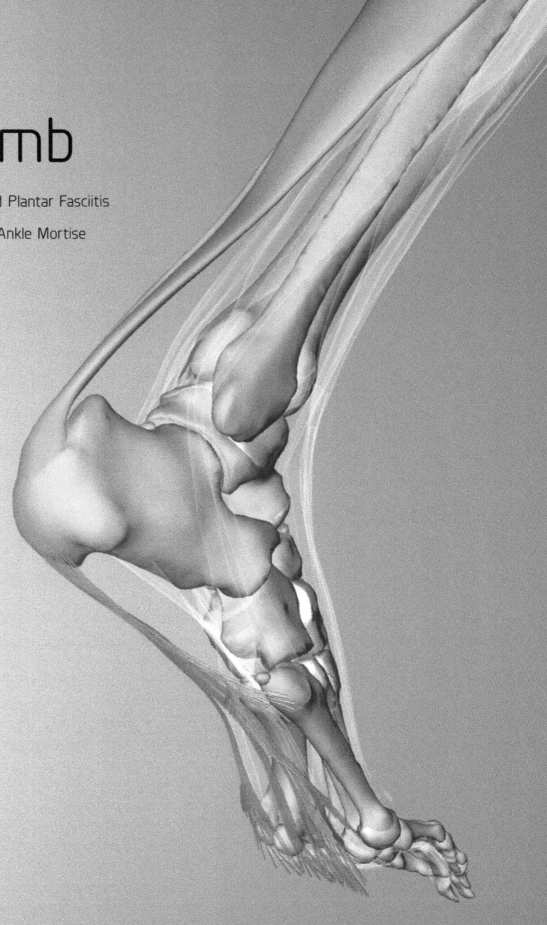

Lower Limb

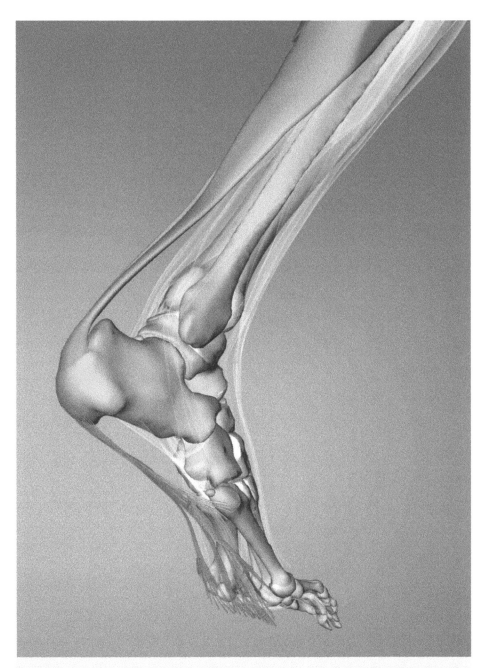

Figure 4.1

There is a continuous line of connection from the gastrocnemius/soleus to the plantar fascia (whose fibrous aponeuroses are shown here in salmon). A lack of resilience anywhere in the chain will restrict ankle dorsiflexion, and may contribute to Achilles tendon irritation or plantar fasciitis.

Ankles bend, ankles straighten. Why is this important? Try walking without bending your ankles. If you have ever attempted to walk in ski boots, you will recognize the awkwardness and stiffness that comes with a loss of ankle motion.

Ankles bend in two sagittal directions – plantarflexion (from the Latin *plantaris flectere*, "sole bent"), and *dorsiflexion* (bent towards the dorsal or upper side of the foot). While plantarflexion gives a powerful push-off to each stride and adds spring to a jump, the complementary motion of dorsiflexion is at least as important. Squatting, kneeling, lunging, running, and landing from a jump all require dorsiflexion, as do many other crucial functions related to our ability to get around and function freely. Dorsiflexion, when lost, limits more than just ankle movement – it limits our overall mobility and adaptability.

There are two main types of structural restrictions that can limit standing dorsiflexion.[1] We will refer to them as Type 1 and Type 2:

- Type 1: Dorsiflexion will be limited if the soft tissue structures on the posterior side of the leg and foot resist lengthening. These structures include the gastrocnemius, soleus, superficial and deep fasciae, the long toe flexors, and the plantar fascia.
- Type 2: Inelastic connective tissues joining the tibia and fibula (such as the extensor retinacula, interosseous membrane and tibiofibular ligaments) can prevent these two bones from normal widening around the wedge-shaped talus (more about this in Chapter 5, *Type 2 Restrictions and the Ankle Mortise*).

These two types of restrictions can occur together, but often one type will be the primary or most obvious restriction. In general, Type 2

---

1 The contributing causes of both types of restrictions can include soft tissue shortening, hardening, or scarring from overuse, postural habit, surgery, or injury, as well as neurological conditions such as cerebral palsy. The contractures from these conditions will usually respond well to the work presented in this book. Restrictions from joint abnormalities or bone spurs are also possible, and although the work described here may be helpful, additional measures and care by other professionals is usually indicated.

is more common when there is very limited dorsiflexion (as in the person on the right in Figure 4.3), though this is variable.

In this chapter, I will begin by discussing a number of ways to work with a Type 1 restriction – to help the soft tissues in the back of the lower limb to lengthen and be as responsive as possible. We will examine Type 2 restrictions – a fixed relationship between the tibia and fibula – in the next chapter.

Dorsiflexion test

We can assess the amount of dorsiflexion available and identify the primary type of restriction by asking our client to do a deep knee bend with parallel feet. Look at the angle of the lower leg in relationship to the foot (Figures 4. 2 and 4.3). How deep can the knee bend go before the available dorsiflexion is used up and the heels have to come off the ground?

In general, the more dorsiflexion, the better, even for people with frontal plane ankle instabilities, such as pronation, supination, or a tendency toward ankle sprains. (Having greater adaptability in the sagittal plane can reduce the lateral forces that cause ankle turns or over-pronation.)

Once you have assessed the amount of dorsiflexion, you will need to determine where to work. Your client will usually be able to direct you to the predominant restriction. At the full limit of dorsiflexion, ask: "What stops you from going further? Where exactly do you feel that?" The most common answers are a stretch or tightness in the back of the calf, sometimes including the sole of the foot (a Type 1 restriction), or a jamming, crunching, or pinching at the anterior fold of the ankle (indicating a Type 2 restriction).[2] We will now look at two techniques that will help address the first type of restriction: shortness in the posterior leg and/or foot.

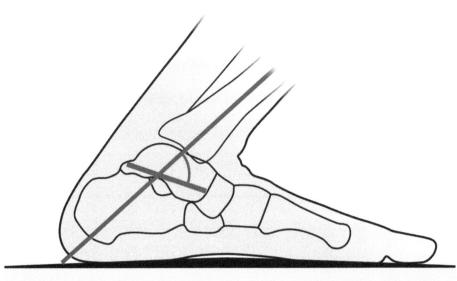

Figure 4.2

Dorsiflexion refers to the angle between the tibia and the talus.

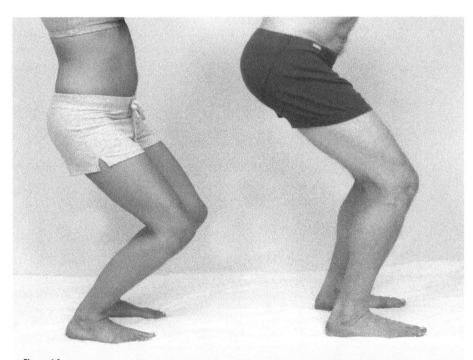

Figure 4.3

In the Dorsiflexion Test, look for the degree of ankle dorsiflexion possible before the heels lift off the floor. In addition to the angle between the foot and the tibia, compensations such as turning the feet out (seen in the person on the left), foot pronation, lifting the arms forward for balance, or leaning forward at the hips (as the person on the right is doing), are all possible signs of limited dorsiflexion.

2 Sometimes clients will report a straining or cramping in the front of the shin, instead of a stretching in the back or jamming sensation in the front. If they seem to be referring to the tibialis anterior area, this is usually related to Type II restriction, which is discussed in Chapter 5. If the more lateral peroneals seem to be the source of the sensation, those will usually respond to direct work at the site of discomfort, combined with active dorsiflexion and plantarflexion, as the peroneals themselves can contribute to limited dorsiflexion (see Figure 4.5).

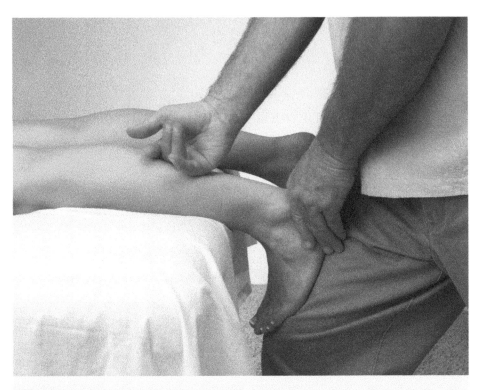

Figure 4.4

Using a soft fist combined with assisted dorsiflexion via the practitioner's leg, in the Gastrocnemius Technique.

Ankle Mobility Techniques

The Soft Fist

Both of the techniques in this chapter use the practitioner's "soft fist" as a tool. This has several advantages over using a palm, fingers, or other parts of the hand as traditionally used in soft-tissue manual therapy:

• Once you are accustomed to using a soft fist, you will find that it allows you to address particular structures and tissue layers with greater specificity and less work, as by keeping your wrist aligned with the metacarpals of your hand, you can transmit pressure with almost no muscular effort.

• The neutral position of the wrist keeps the carpal tunnel open, preventing the neurovascular compression and overuse injuries that can accompany frequent or habitual wrist extension.

The keys to a sensitive, comfortable, soft fist are to keep your wrist straight, your hand open, and let the knuckles of the middle fingers do the work.

Gastrocnemius/Soleus Technique

As the strongest and largest muscle group on the back of the leg, the gastrocnemius/soleus complex is the most obvious place to work when you see limited dorsiflexion. Injuries or strains of the gastrocnemius and soleus are common, especially with activities such as racquet sports, basketball, skiing, or running. Tissue shortening resulting from injury, or simply from normal use, can reduce the ankle's ability to dorsiflex.

With your client prone and with his or her feet off the end of the table, use your soft fist to anchor the stocking-like outer layers of fascia (the superficial and crural fasciae). We will work with one layer at a time, releasing each before going deeper. Ask your client for slow, deliberate ankle movement (plantar- and dorsiflexion). Use the lengthening effects of dorsiflexion to release any shortened or tighter lines of tissue (Figure 4.4), as you apply a slight cephalad (head-ward) resistance to the tissues under your touch.

Although your touch will slide slightly, let your client's active ankle dorsiflexion initiate and pace your movement. Once you have felt the outer layers lengthen, feel into the deeper Achilles tendon and the conjoined heads of the gastrocnemius and soleus itself. Continue the active movement, as you gradually work deeper on each pass. Check in frequently with your client about the pace and depth of this movement. As postural muscles that are always engaged when standing, the gastrocnemius complex can be particularly tender, especially at deeper levels.

Since the long toe flexors can also restrict dorsiflexion, ask for active toe extension in combination with dorsiflexion. This lengthens and structurally differentiates the flexor hallicus longus and flexor digitorum longus from each other, and from their neighbors. Since these are

---

Key points: Gastrocnemius/Soleus Technique

Indications include:
- Type I dorsiflexion restriction.
- Achilles Tendon or calf pain.
- Plantar Fasciitis.

Purpose
- Increase layer differentiation and tissue adaptability.
- Prepare outer layers of the lower leg for deeper work.

Instructions
- Use gentle friction and tension to feel for and release any restrictions in outer layers of the lower leg.

Movements
- Active dorsiflexion.

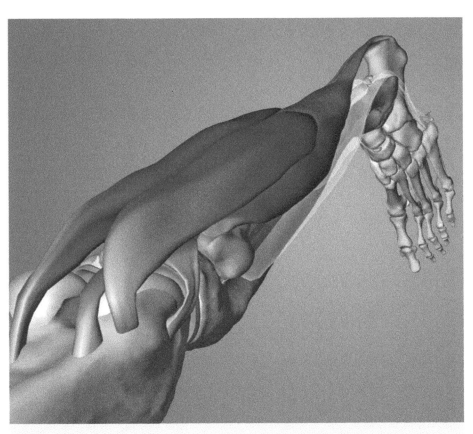

Figure 4.5

Use the Gastrocnemius Technique all the way to the gastrocnemii origins on the posterior side of the distal femur (left edge of image). Also visible in this view are the peroneus longus and brevis (transparent), which like the gastrocnemius/soleus complex, can also limit dorsiflexion.

the deepest structures in the calf, this makes this technique even more effective.

As long as your client is comfortable and able to relax into the work, you can incorporate an additional measure of passive gastrocnemius stretch with your leg (Figure 4.4). Use your soft fist or gentle finger pressure to work all the way to the proximal origins of the medial and lateral gastrocnemius heads on the posterior femur (Figure 4.5), being cautious around the nerves in the popliteal fossa at the back of the knee.

Plantar Fascia Technique

See video of the Plantar Fascia Technique at http://advanced-trainings.com/v/la05.html

The sole of the foot has alternating layers of broad connective tissue strata, short strong muscles, and long cord-like tendons and ligaments. Shortness in any of these layers can limit dorsiflexion through their collective continuity with the gastrocnemius/soleus complex, as seen in Figure 4.1. The plantar fascia is a strong, fibrous layer covering the entire sole, lying superficial to the short toe flexors and just deep to the subcutaneous fat of the heel (Figure 4.7). Plantar fasciitis is a common inflammatory condition of this layer, characterized by heel and mid-foot pain, and most often with point tenderness at the plantar fascia's insertion on the distal and inferior surfaces of the calcaneus. Contributive factors include improper foot and leg biomechanics, overuse, and fascial shortness in the calf or hamstrings.

Direct work with the plantar surface of the foot, including the plantar fascia, is indicated when clients report a stretch or pain in the sole with the Dorsiflexion Test. Local plantar pain, cramping, and stiffness are also indications for using this technique, as is plantar fasciitis.

Because plantar fasciitis involves tissue inflammation, the conventional wisdom is to avoid working directly on the most painful areas

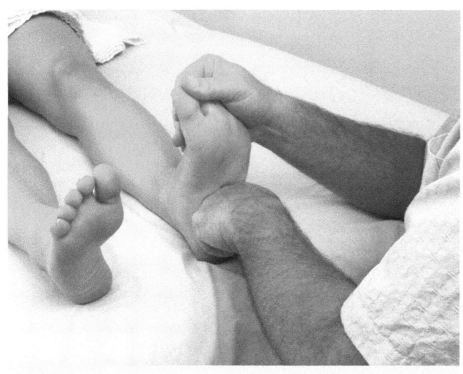

Figure 4.6
The Plantar Fascia Technique combines the soft fist with active or passive toe extension. In Plantar Fasciitis, avoid direct pressure on the most tender areas so as not to further aggravate the inflammation. Instead, lengthen and release the tissue distal to the inflamed points.

(usually the proximal attachments on the calcaneus). Although some practitioners report good results by carefully working directly on the most painful areas, the most cautious approach would be to lengthen, release, and ease the entire plantar surface around (rather than at) the points of greatest tenderness. If you are not getting the results you want from the indirect approach, you might want to discuss using a direct approach with your client, making sure he or she is aware of the risk of experiencing increased inflammation afterwards as a possible result of working directly on the inflamed tissues. If your client reports less discomfort in the days after your session, even if the relief was transitory, you are on track. If there was a worsening of the symptoms, or if no change was evident afterwards, return to working globally rather than locally.

"Recalcitrant", or stubborn, plantar fasciitis is treated surgically by "releasing" (partially severing) the plantar fascia, with the aim of relieving the strain on the inflamed attachments. Our intention is similar, though our methods are different – instead of severing the fascia, feel for a lengthening release in both of the techniques described here. In combination with hamstring or peroneal work, clients often show tangible improvements in the degree of plantar tenderness within one or two sessions. A longer series of sessions is often necessary for chronic sufferers, as is regular stretching, a change in usage patterns, and improved biomechanics (via methods like structural integration, orthotics, movement instruction, or improved footwear).

To work with the plantar fascia, we use the middle knuckles of a soft fist (Figure 4.6). As in the Gastrocnemius Technique, start with the superficial layers, releasing first the skin, then the subcutaneous layers, then the plantar fascia. Use active or passive toe extension to move the tissue layers under your touch. Be sensitive, thorough, and slow. Remember, you are releasing your

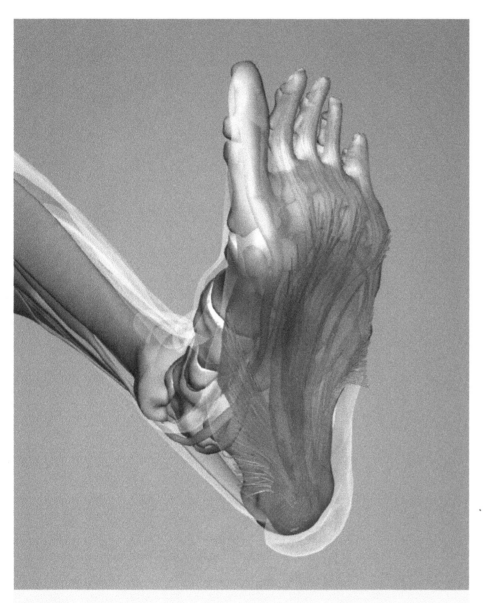

Figure 4.7

The plantar fascia is a broad layer of tough connective tissue covering the sole of the foot. Within it are bands of mostly longitudinal fibers (the plantar aponeuroses, in orange). The proximal end of the plantar fascia lies deep to the thick calcaneal fat pad (transparent).

Key points: Plantar Fascia Technique

Indications include:

- Restricted dorsiflexion or toe extension.
- Type I dorsiflexion restriction.
- Plantar fasciitis, pain, stiffness, or cramping.

Purpose

- Increase differentiation and adaptability of plantar fascial layers.

Instructions

- Beginning with superficial fascial layers of the foot, use slow gliding of a soft fist or knuckle, in combination with active or passive movement.
- Feel for tissue lengthening on eccentric (dorsiflexion or toe extension) phase.
- Work cautiously with areas of possible inflammation, noting response between sessions to gauge appropriateness of direct work.

Movements

- Active or passive dorsiflexion and toe extension.

client's nervous system as well as their connective tissue, so be sure to allow time for your client to breathe, release, and relax into the work.

The techniques covered in this section serve as ideal preparation for the deeper work described in the next chapter, where our focus will be on the second type of dorsiflexion restriction: a fixation of the tibia and fibula around the talus.

Picture credits

Figures 4.1, 4.5 and 4.7 courtesy Primal Pictures.
Figures 4.2, 4.3, 4.4 and 4.6 courtesy Advanced-Trainings.com.

Study Guide

Type 1 Ankle Restrictions and Plantar Fasciitis

1 The text states that in the Dorsiflexion Test, a Type 1 ankle restriction will usually be felt in:

a the anterior calf
b the ankle bones
c interosseous membrane
d the posterior calf

2 As stated in the text, some of the most logical structures to work in a Type 1 ankle restriction are:

a the gastrocnemius/soleus complex
b the bones of the ankle joint
c the tibialis anterior and long toe flexors
d the interosseous membrane and tibiofibular ligaments

3 In the Dorsiflexion Test, the text states that a Type 2 ankle restriction will typically be felt:

a in the posterior calf
b in the anterior ankle crease
c in the plantar fascia
d behind the knee

4 The text states that when performing the Gastrocnemius/Soleus Technique, use caution to avoid compressing the nerves at:

a the cleft between the heads of the gastrocnemius
b the medial edge of the soleus
c the posterior knee
d the Achilles tendon attachments

5 When working with plantar fasciitis the text recommends avoiding working directly on the most painful areas, which are most often the:

a distal plantar fascia attachments
b midfoot plantar fascia
c proximal plantar fascia attachments
d fat pad of the heel

For Answer Keys, visit www.Advanced-Trainings.com/v1key/

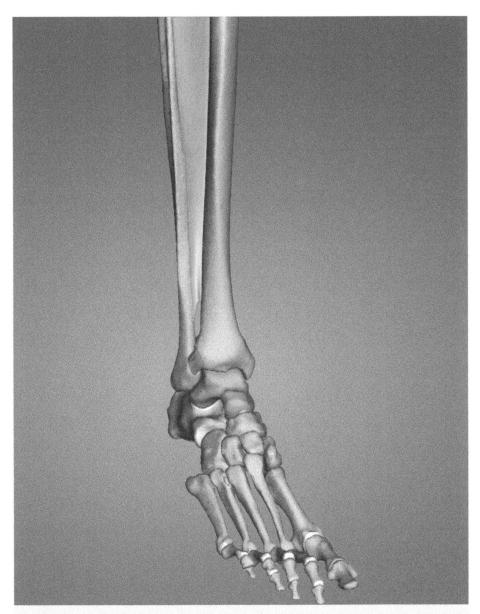

Figure 5.1

The tibia and fibula form a fork-like mortise around the talus bone (orange), giving the ankle both stability and adaptability. When the interosseous membrane and tibiofibular ligaments (violet) don't allow normal resilience and spring in the ankle mortise, dorsiflexion will be limited.

For us bipeds, upright movement demands a delicate balance of joint mobility and stability. Ankles provide both: their mobility allows us to walk, run, jump, skip and hop; and their inherent stability supports and balances the considerable weight of the rest of the body through all the movements the ankles allow.

The bones of the ankles have the qualities of mobility and stability built in. The solidly constructed tibia transmits the body's weight to the talus, the uppermost bone of the foot (Figure 5.1). The smaller fibula rides alongside the tibia, providing an added dimension of stability by wrapping around the talus in a fork-like mortise-and-tenon joint. Except that, unlike a cabinetmaker's hardwood mortise, this living joint walks, runs, dances, skateboards, stands on tiptoe, plays tennis, etc. It is the talus' unique shape that allows the ankle's solidity and mobility to coexist. Examining the talus, we see that its upper articular surface (the trochlea or tibial plafond) is slightly wedge-shaped (Figure 5.2). This wedge is the tenon that fits inside the mortise formed by the distal ends of the tibia and fibula. The narrowest part of the wedge is the posterior plafond[1] – the portion that lies between the tibia and fibula in plantarflexion. This narrowness gives the articulation more play and mobility in plantarflexion, allowing the foot to adapt to uneven surfaces when landing with the midfoot.[2] Conversely, in dorsiflexion the widest part of the wedge-shaped talus completely fills the gap between the tibia and fibula, firming up the ankle joint and giving bony solidity to the push-off phase, which is when stability is most needed.

Even when completely dorsiflexed, this form-closed joint is not rigid, at least ideally. In normal function, the connective tissues joining tibia and fibula actually permit some springiness between

---

1 For word-buffs, a "plafond" is an ornately decorated ceiling. It originates from the French plat "flat" + fond "bottom, base." Accordingly, the tibial plafond could be thought of as both an ornate, wedge-shaped ceiling for the talus, and a base for the tibia above it.

2 In contrast to an adaptable landing with the mid-foot, a thumping heel-strike is harder and less accommodating, due in part to the wider part of the talus being wedged between the malleoli of the tibia and fibula. The timing of the knee's extension in the gait cycle plays a large role in determining which part of the foot contacts the ground first.

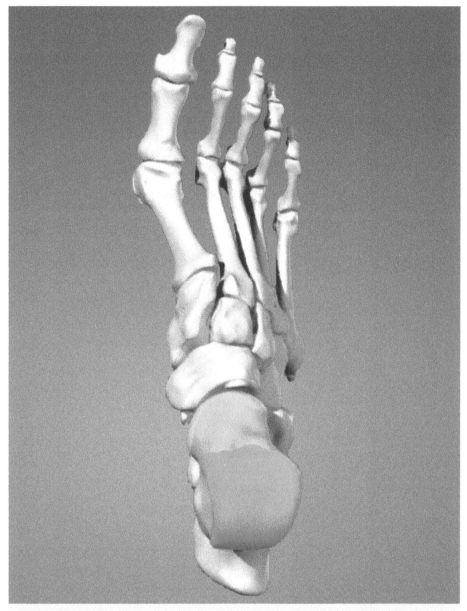

Figure 5.2

The talus (orange) has a superior articular surface (darker orange) which is 5–6 mm wider anteriorly, giving it a wedged shape. The widest part of the wedge moves between the tibia and fibula in dorsiflexion.

these two bones, allowing an elastic firmness to their hold on the talus. When this slight elasticity in the connective tissues is lost (through hardening due to injury, overuse, or inefficient biomechanics), the tibia and fibula act more like a clamp than a spring (Figure 5.3). When particularly fixed, this inelasticity stops the talus before full dorsiflexion is reached, limiting the range of dorsiflexion. Our clients often experience this restriction as a jamming or pinching sensation in the front of the ankle during dorsiflexion.

We are referring to this clamping around the talus as a "Type 2" dorsiflexion restriction (Type 1 being related to shortness in the tissues of the posterior leg and plantar surface of the foot). In Chapter 4 we discussed ways to assess these two types of restrictions, and to work with Type I restrictions. In this chapter, we'll look at ways to restore lost dorsiflexion by insuring adaptability of the tibia and fibula around the wedge of the talus.

Retinacula Technique

The crural fascia (or fascia cruris, cruris meaning "leg") is a thick membranous wrapping around the lower leg. Like built-in support hose the crural fascia provides the reinforcement, encasing, and undergirding needed by the leg's powerful structures. Releasing this layer helps prepare for the deeper work we'll do with the ankle mortise itself.

Within the crural fascia are the retinacula, fibrous bands at places of particular strain. Deep to the retinacula, cord-like tendons round the corner of the ankle, on their way from their origins in the leg to their attachments in the foot (Figure 5.4). The ankle is a busy place – with the exception of a few thigh muscles that just make it past the knee, all lower leg muscles cross the ankle into the foot. With the entire force of standing and locomotion being transmitted across the ankle, the restraining structures here

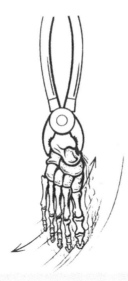

Figure 5.3
When adaptability between the tibia and fibula is lost, the widest part of the talus gets squeezed during dorsiflexion.

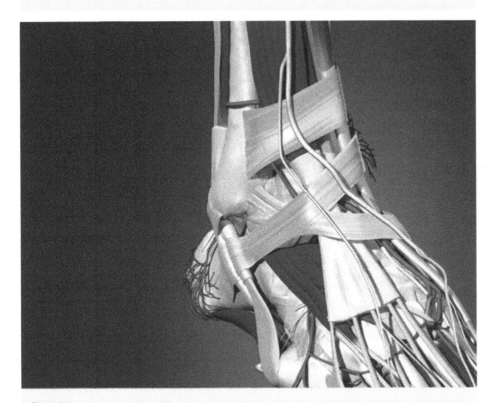

Figure 5.4
The retinacula are fibrous bands within the crural fascia. When restricted, they can irritate bursa (light blue), or limit the adaptability needed for full ankle range.

are thick, resilient, and dense – which is fine, except when they do their restraining too well. Retinacula that are too tight can irritate the bursa underneath them. They can also limit the adaptability of the ankle by binding the tendons they overlie, or by restricting the necessary spreading of the tibia and fibula around the talus.

To ensure adaptability of the crural fascia and the retinacula, use the ends of your curled fingers to feel for and release any restrictions in these outer layers. Using the tips of your nails, push proximally, rather than pulling distally. Feel for the fibrous layers of fascia just under the skin (Figures 5.5 and 5.6). Imagine pushing up your client's tight-but-sagging socks. The pressure is firm; your pace is slow and patient. Rather than gliding over the skin, take time to feel for the tough layers just deep to the dermis. Feel for fibrous banding here, and for any adhesion to the layers below. Ask for slow, active dorsiflexion and plantarflexion. Apply sensitive but firm proximal pressure to these areas and wait for release. Work the crural fascia of the entire lower half of the leg, as well as the retinacula of the ankle and the fascia dorsalis pedis of the instep (Figure 5.6).

Key points: Retinacula Technique

Indications include:
- Type 2 dorsiflexion restriction.
- Bursa irritation or nerve pain at the ankle.

Purpose
- Increase layer differentiation and tissue adaptability.
- Prepare outer layers of lower leg for deeper work.

Instructions
- Use gentle friction and tension to feel for and release any restrictions in outer layers of lower leg.

Movements
- Active dorsiflexion.

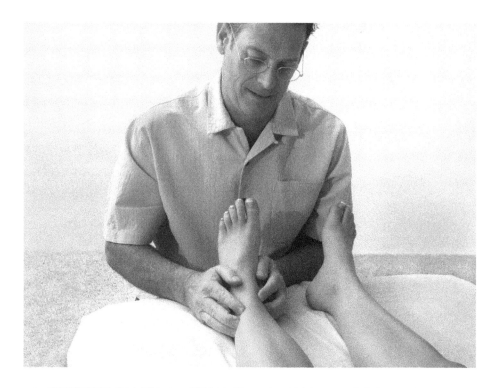

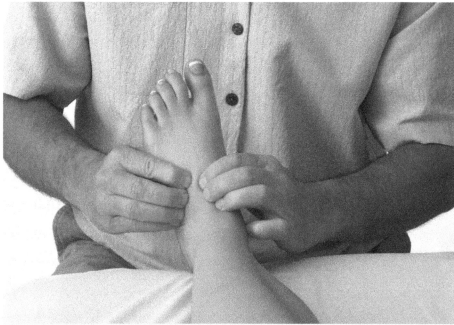

Figures 5.5/5.6

For the Crural Fascia/Retinacula Technique, use the tips of your curled fingers, with just a bit of fingernail, to feel for and release restricted areas in the crural fascia.

Tibialis Anterior Technique

Although the tibialis anterior muscle won't usually restrict ankle dorsiflexion directly, we include it in our protocol here as preparation for the Interosseous Membrane Technique. The tibialis anterior and the long toe extensors that lie deep to it must be released before work with the deepest interosseous layer is comfortable for the client. Additionally, some clients will feel discomfort or cramping in the tibialis anterior region with the Dorsiflexion Test (Chapter 4). This usually accompanies a Type II dorsiflexion restriction (related to tibia/fibula mortise restrictions, rather than shortened ankle plantarflexors).

Using a soft fist or the flat of your forearm, slowly glide along the length of the tibialis anterior, encouraging length and tissue elasticity as your client actively dorsiflexes and plantarflexes the ankle. Feel for release, particularly on the eccentric (plantarflexion) phase. Once the outer layers have been worked, repeat the technique, adding

Key points: Tibialis Anterior Technique

Indications include:
- Restricted plantarflexion or toe flexion.
- Shin splints.
- Type 2 dorsiflexion restriction (preparation).

Purpose
- Increase myofascial differentiation and adaptability of the anterior lower leg.
- Tissue preparation for the Interosseous Membrane Technique.

Instructions
- Use slow gliding of a soft fist or forearm on the myofascia of anterior lower leg, feeling for tissue lengthening on eccentric (plantarflexion or toe flexion) phase.

Movements
- Active ankle plantarflexion and dorsiflexion; active toe flexion and extension.

active toe flexion and extension to access and release the deeper extensor digitorum longus and extensor hallucis longus (Figure 5.7).

Although direction of work (proximal to distal, or the reverse) is usually not a crucial factor in our approach, you'll often find that one direction feels more effective to you and to the client. As an experiment, check both directions, and get descriptive feedback about the difference.

Interosseous Membrane Technique

Remember that the tibia and fibula will limit dorsiflexion if they can't spread slightly around the widest part of the talar wedge. The deepest and strongest structures restricting this widening are the interosseous membrane and its associated tibiofibular ligaments.

Even after preparing the outer layers of the lower leg with the two preceding techniques, we aren't able to directly touch the deep interosseous membrane of the leg, at least not comfortably. To work the membrane, we can use the fibula as a convenient handle to laterally stretch the tough membrane and ligaments that join it to the tibia. *Fibula* is Latin for "brooch," after its resemblance (along with the tibia) to a clasp, with the fibula being the pin. (More ideas for working with the fibula are explored in Chapter 6.) The Interosseous Membrane Technique opens the clasp, allowing more room for the talus to move.

Use the knuckles of both soft fists to pull on the medial side of the fibula, using your weight rather than muscular strength (Figures 5.8 and 5.9). Ask your client for full dorsiflexion, pausing at the end range of the movement so that the widest part of the talar wedge can assist you in widening the tibial/fibular space. Your pressure is quite firm, but still comfortable for your client. The strong interosseous structures respond slowly, so be sure to wait long enough to feel the subtle release and widening of the fibula away from

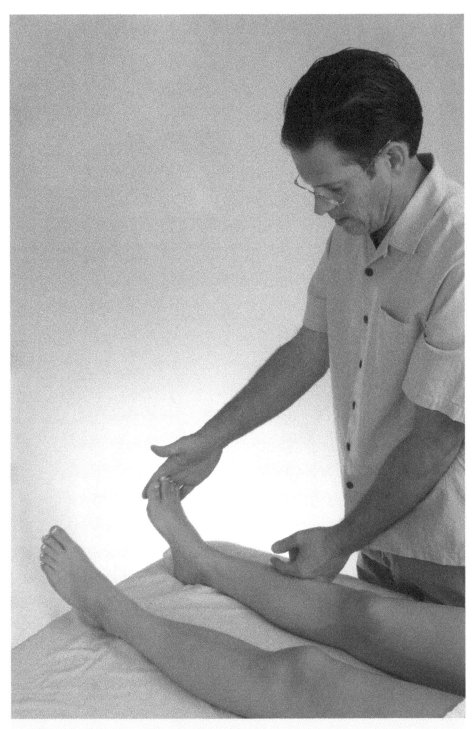

Figure 5.7

Using a soft fist combined with active dorsiflexion in the Tibialis Anterior Technique.

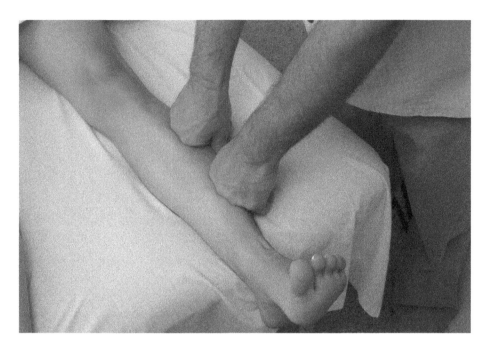

the tibia. It can be helpful to imagine unrolling the two bones of the lower leg like the two parts of a scroll. There is, in fact, a small amount of external fibular rotation with dorsiflexion (1) and adding this dimension to your lower leg work can increase its effectiveness.

Once you've felt the fibula respond, shift your knuckles to a new place, repeating this technique along the entire length of the fibula, particularly at the distal end, where the tibiofibular ligaments are located.

After working the first leg, ask your client to stand and walk for a few steps, comparing the sensations of the worked and un-worked legs. Often the difference in mobility and stability will be profound. Ask your client to repeat this comparison again after working the second leg.

Key points: Interosseous Membrane Technique

Indications include:
- Type 2 dorsiflexion restriction.

Purpose
- Increase resilient adaptability between the fibula and tibia.

Instructions
- Use knuckles of soft fist to apply lateral pressure on the fibula, in combination with active.
- Dorsiflexion. Wait for slight lateral yielding of fibula.

Movements
- Active dorsiflexion.

Figures 5.8/5.9

The Interosseous Membrane Technique. After preparing the outer layers of the lower leg, use the knuckles of a soft fist to encourage the fibula to release laterally, giving more room for the talus. Use your client's active dorsiflexion to bring the widest part of the talus between the tibia and fibula, augmenting the release.

Over-pronation and hypermobility

Our overall intention with these techniques is to relieve any dorsiflexion restrictions by ensuring that the fibula and tibia can spring and widen slightly around the wedge-shape talus, particularly in full dorsiflexion. But what about ankles that already seem too mobile, such as in over-pronation patterns, or unstable ankles that twist easily?

In theory, both over-pronation and ankle sprains can cause laxity in the talar mortis. However, in practice, you'll see many clients with those issues who also have limited dorsiflexion at the talar/tibial joint. In the Dorsiflexion Test, you'll frequently see people using a combination of foot pronation, eversion, and external tibial rotation when talar dorsiflexion is limited. Similarly, losing the front/back adaptability that dorsiflexion provides can increase lateral forces on the ankle, leading to greater vulnerability to ankle turning and rolling.

This is not to say that ankle hypermobility does not exist. There are cases where there is clearly too much laxity between the tibia and fibula, usually as the result of congenital conditions or from an unhealed or serious injury. These clients can benefit from a referral to an orthopedist or rehabilitation specialist. Empirically, we've found that in even these cases, and certainly in the majority of people, whenever any dorsiflexion restrictions are released, clients experience improvement in balance, stability, and less tendency towards over-pronation, even when there is also an apparent side-to-side hypermobility.

Reference

[1] Forst, J. et al. (1993) "Effect of upper tibial osteotomy on fibula movement and ankle joint motion." Archives of Orthopaedic and Trauma Surgery. 112, no. 5. p. 239–242.

Figure credits

Figures 5.1 and 5.4 courtesy Primal Pictures.
Figure 5.2: Source courtesy Primal Pictures.
Figure 5.3 courtesy Eric Franklin, originator of the Franklin Method (www.franklin-method.com).
Figures 5.5–5.9 courtesy Advanced-Trainings.com.

Study Guide

Type 2 Restrictions and the Ankle Mortise

1 **Dorsiflexion is affected by the tarsal's plafond being wider:**

a Anteriorly
b Posteriorly
c Laterally
d Medially

2 **This helps the ankle joint be more adaptable in:**

a Dorsiflexion
b Plantarflexion
c Pronation
d Supination

3 **In a Type 2 restriction, dorsiflexion is most directly limited by:**

a Shortened or tight posterior leg structures
b Shortened or tight anterior leg structures
c Lack of spring between the tibia and talus
d Lack of spring between the tibia and fibula

4 **Of the following, which does the chapter say is the strongest structure that limits tibia/fibula widening?**

a Tibialis anterior
b Interosseous membrane
c Soleus
d Fascia cruris

5 **The chapter states that the limited dorsiflexion will often be seen together with:**

a Over pronation
b Eversion
c Either of the above
d None of the above

For Answer Keys, visit www.Advanced-Trainings.com/v1key/

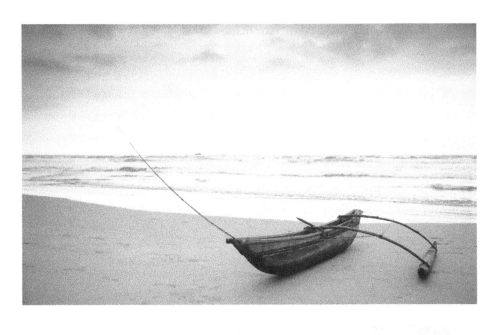

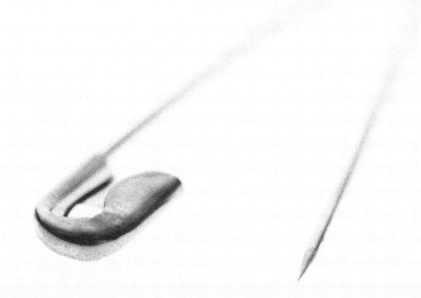

Figures 6.1/6.2

Analogies used to describe the fibula's function include a canoe's outrigger and a safety pin. "Fibula" means pin or clasp.

The fibula gets short shrift. Often overlooked and underrated as a mere "outrigger" or companion bone to the tibia, the fibula is one of the body's many structures that help balance the exquisitely paradoxical qualities of stability and adaptability. As such, fibular mobility plays an important role in both normal movement and in recovery from ankle injuries (of which there are an estimated 25,000 per day in the US alone) (1). Yet, paradoxically, many hands-on practitioners pay little attention to the fibula.

While modern Romance languages refer to the fibula as the "peroneal bone" (from the Greek word for "pin"), English texts have used the Latin word *fibula* for about 300 years, which also represents the pin of a brooch, buckle, or clasp. It is this clasp-like relationship of the fibula with the tibia – much like the two sides of a safety pin (Figures 6.1 & 6.2) – which helps the ankle mortise (Figure 6.3) to hold the foot's talus bone in a springy but firm grip at the distal tibiofibular joint. It is this joint's combination of resilience and firmness that stabilizes the ankle hinge enough that it can support our weight, while being free enough to swing wide in plantar- and dorsiflexion.

Differing perspectives on ankle injuries

It is the ankle's strong ligaments that give it the adaptability to spring back (in most cases) when stressed. When forces are too great for the ligaments, they can slightly, partially, or completely tear; these are known as Grade I, II, or III sprains, respectively. The tibia, fibula, and talus can also fracture in more severe injuries. Ankle injuries of all severities involve damage to the joint capsules, tendons, retinacula, and fascial layers of the lower leg, which are often

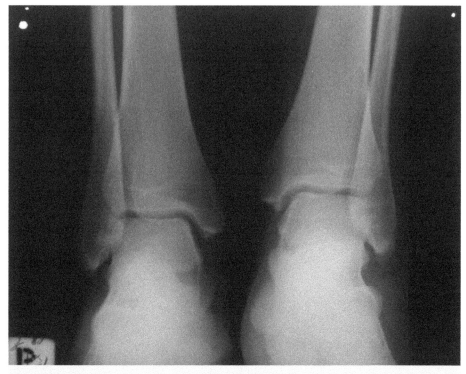

Figure 6.3

An X-ray figure of the ankle mortise – the fibula and tibia's clasp-like relationship with the foot's talus bone. Balanced bony mobility is crucial to protect the thin articular surfaces from stress and degeneration.

responsible for much of an injury's swelling, pain, and discoloration. Injury to these connective tissue structures is more common than serious ligamentous or bone damage.

While most sources agree that some of the ankle's connective tissues can recover from minor to moderate injuries relatively quickly, the conventional view is that if the ligaments themselves are compromised, recovery for moderate to severe sprains can take anywhere from six weeks to one year. This timeline is quoted by the American Academy of Orthopaedic Surgeons, which also advises that "patience and learning to cope with an injury is essential to recovery" (2). And other sources say it may take even longer – one study says that as many as 30 percent of those who injure their ankles still have pain after one year (3).

However, views vary widely on which tissues are being injured, and how long the recovery should take. A vocal minority of sports rehabilitation specialists claim that true ligamentous damage is far less common than is often assumed. This point of view asserts that by encouraging gentle movement and increased blood flow soon after a moderate injury (via manipulation, traction, as well as through passive and active movements), ankle recovery times can be significantly shorter than with conventional treatments (4). Although proponents of this view could be criticized for relying on dramatic anecdotes and empirical evidence rather than on clinical research, the conventional protocol of rest, ice, compression, and elevation (or RICE), despite being widely used and extensively studied, has largely failed to be proven effective in controlled clinical trials (5). In addition, most schools of thought now favor the use of gentle motion as soon as possible following an injury, rather than advising the patient to engage in prolonged rest or immobilization of the limb. (Of course, to be prudent, serious ankle injuries should be evaluated by a qualified rehabilitation specialist – typically for

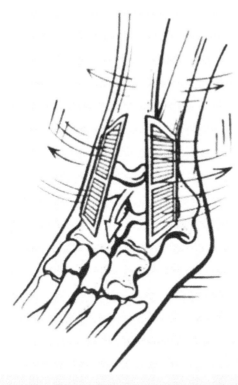

Figure 6.4

Fibular rotation with ankle movement varies between individuals, leading to conflicting biomechanical models. Franklin's imaginative swinging door analogy links external fibular motion with dorsiflexion, but most other sources cite the opposite (Figure 6.5.) (The anterior tibiofibular ligament and interosseous membrane are also shown).

swelling, discoloration, deformity, tenderness, and range of motion – before assuming that ligament compromise is or isn't present.)

Whichever view ultimately prevails, whether recovery can happen fast or needs more time, and whether manipulation or rest is indicated in the acute phase, an unresolved injury puts the ankle more at risk for problems like prolonged discomfort, chronic disability, early arthritis, and especially reinjury. In fact, according to one large-scale study, the only consistent risk factor for injuring an ankle is having suffered a prior sprain, both for physically active people and for individuals who are less so (6). Although an exhaustive discussion about ankle injuries and the various approaches used to treat them is beyond our current scope, you can find references to other relevant sections in this book and other sources of information regarding ankle injuries at the end of this chapter.

Restoring fibular mobility

One of the most effective ways we can contribute to the prevention and recovery of ankle injuries is by restoring balanced fibular mobility. To understand fibular motion, we need to review the shape of the talus, the top bone in the foot. The superior articular surface of the talus, where it lies within the fork-like mortise formed by the tibia and fibula (Figure 6.3), is wider anteriorly than posteriorly. As this wider part of the wedge-shaped talus rolls between the tibia and fibula in dorsiflexion, these two bones spread apart slightly (Figure 6.5). Normally, this lateral translation is 3–5 millimeters, and is limited by the stretch of the interosseous and tibiofibular ligaments, which give this joint its spring. This is also the mechanism that explains why squeezing the lateral and medial malleoli together on a cadaver results in foot plantarflexion; this does not typically happen with living bodies, prevented by the leg muscles' postural resting tone (7).

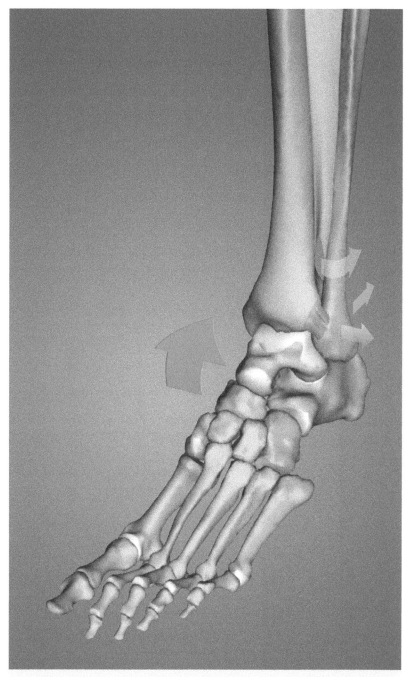

Figure 6.5

In this model, with ankle dorsiflexion (blue arrow), the fibula normally rotates (yellow arrow), glides posteriorly (green), and spreads laterally away from the tibia (pink arrow). Whichever model is used, when these small fibular motions are restricted, ankle motion and adaptability is impaired.

In addition to its lateral translation and posterior glide, the fibula also rotates with ankle movement (Figure 6.4). There is significant disagreement about how fibular rotation is coupled with ankle movement. Although Franklin (Figure 6.4) and Kapandji (8) describe the opposite, most of the other references surveyed for this chapter indicate that the fibula rotates externally when the ankle dorsiflexes. This lack of consistency between otherwise credible sources might be due to the fact that fibular motion actually varies in different people. One 2008 study assessing cadavers' fibular motion (n = 20) showed "no consistent pattern for rotation" coupled with dorsiflexion; some specimens rotated externally, while others rotated internally (9). There is also little agreement on the amount of fibular rotation considered normal, with cited measurements ranging from two degrees (10) to 30 degrees (11) of malleolus rotation.

However, whether internal or external, large or small, there is common agreement that some fibular rotation is an essential part of normal ankle function. Not only does fibular mobility add adaptability to this important joint, but it also helps the talus remain in close contact with the ankle mortise throughout its dorsiflexion/plantarflexion range. This close but pliable contact is crucial for even load distribution (12) and balanced stability/adaptability in standing and in gait. Put another way, unimpaired fibula translation and rotation gives functional resilience, and it also helps protect the thin layer of articular cartilage in the ankle bones from undue stress, damage, and degeneration (13).

Ideas for freeing the talus by working with the retinacula and interosseous membrane were covered in Chapter 5. In this chapter, I will describe two techniques that can be very effective for keeping the fibula mobile and for recovering lost fibular adaptability – whether from injury, habitual movement patterns, or activity.

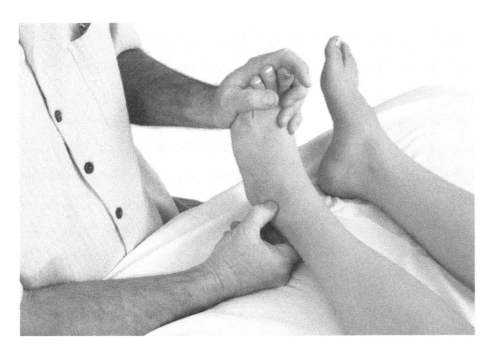

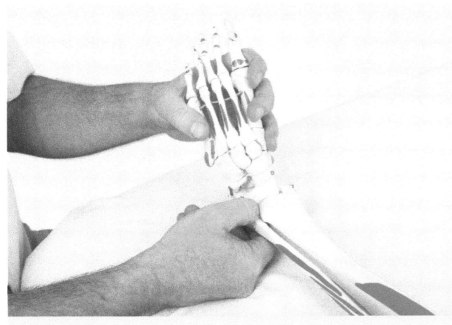

Figures 6.6/6.7

The Distal Tibiofibular Joint Technique combines passive dorsiflexion with pressure into the cleft between the tibia and fibula to restore lateral movement of the fibula.

Techniques for restoring fibular mobility

Distal Tibiofibular Joint Technique

See video of the
Distal Tibofibular
Joint Technique at
http://advanced-
trainings.com/v/
ld08.html

At their lower end, the fibula and tibia join at the distal tibiofibular joint (also known as the tibiofibular syndesmosis). This stiff articulation is bound together by tough, pearly ligaments in front (the anterior tibiofibular ligament, Figure 6.8), in back (the posterior tibiofibular ligament, not pictured), and between the bones (the interosseous ligament, also not pictured). As discussed above, a small amount of springy adaptability in the tibiofibular joint is important for balanced functioning of the ankle, especially for full dorsiflexion, so this technique is useful whenever ankle dorsiflexion is limited.

To begin, feel for the gap between the distal end of the tibia and fibula with your thumb (Figures 6.6 and 6.7) or another tool. Once you have located this fissure between the bones (it is often more lateral than you think), bring your client's ankle into passive dorsiflexion. When the distal end of the fibula is mobile, this fissure will open up or deepen slightly with your passive dorsiflexion, as the wider anterior part of the wedge-shaped talus pushes the fibula laterally. If you don't feel this slight gapping or softening between the bones, continue to apply firm but gentle pressure here, in combination with the passive dorsiflexion. There should be no pain or discomfort; be precise, but not sharp or pointed with your touch. Wait for the joint to respond, as indicated by a slight softening or lateral translation of the fibula. This may take 30–90 seconds.

While you are here, you can use a similar hand position to assess and address anterior/posterior fibular glide. Feel for evenness of fibular mobility at its distal end by stabilizing the tibia's medial malleolus with your medial hand (not pictured),

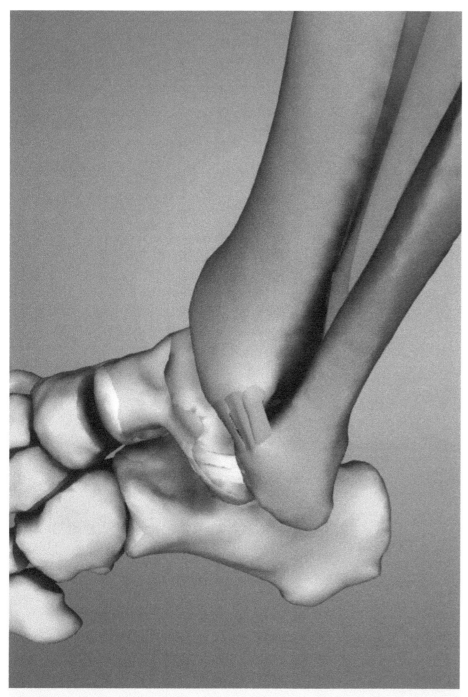

Figure 6.8
The Distal Tibiofibular Joint Technique combines passive dorsiflexion with pressure into the cleft between the tibia and fibula to restore lateral movement of the fibula.

and using a thumb pad or other broad tool to push the fibula's lateral malleolus posteriorly, feeling for the quality and amount of gliding motion. Compare this to pulling the malleolus anteriorly. You can also use your thenar eminence or palm to check for superior glide of the fibula by gently pushing upwards on the underside of the lateral malleolus. Pressure in this direction, in combination with a bit of posterior glide, often brings relief after an ankle inversion injury, as these injuries frequently displace the fibula anteriorly in relationship to the tibia (14).

In working with any of these gliding motions, your grip is firm but comfortable. Feel bone rather than soft tissue, sensing for a small yielding in each direction (in most people, approximately 1–3 millimeters), as you compare anterior with posterior movement. As long as there is no pain, lean into the more restricted direction, and wait for a release.

With any of these techniques, pain with a larger amount of passive fibular motion than observed on the contralateral ankle may indicate ligamentous damage. In these cases, you can be helpful by very gently working the larger area around the joint, without causing any pain. With ligament damage, your intention would be to encourage

Key points: Distal Tibiofibular Joint Technique

Indications include:
- Type 2 dorsiflexion restriction.

Purpose
- Restore lost resilience and adaptability between fibula and tibia.

Instructions
- Sink into the fissure between tibia and fibula. Use gentle but firm pressure to encourage a slight widening of this fissure with dorsiflexion.

Movements
- Active and passive dorsiflexion.

subtle mobility and circulation, rather than trying to release bigger mobility restrictions using deeper pressure, which is more appropriate in working with scarred tissues or restricted joints. Referral to a rehabilitation specialist may also be indicated.

Fibular Head Technique

The fibula does not have just one end. Although its distal joint takes the brunt of most activities, your work will be more comprehensive if you include the proximal end of the fibula when you address ankle issues. The proximal end of the fibula articulates with the tibia via a synovial joint, which allows a small amount of gliding and rotation. In addition to it being a different kind of joint from the firm distal syndesmosis, the proximal joint has smoother articular surfaces than the stiffer distal juncture, and is thus better suited for gliding and translation. Even though the proximal joint is a more mobile structure, in biomechanical testing, it usually moves less than the sturdier distal joint, reflecting the much greater forces that are at work on the distal end.

With your client's knee up (to slacken the biceps femoris, which could otherwise immobilize the fibula), begin by finding a comfortable grip on the proximal head of the fibula (Figure 6.9). Check with your client or patient to make sure you are not pressing on the common peroneal nerve where it passes just behind the fibular head (Figure 6.10). In contrast to the firm, subtle movement of the distal end, the synovial joint of the proximal head will have a looser glide to it, characterized by a distinct start and stop to its mobile range. Check for front/back fibular mobility against the tibia. As with the lower end, balance the proximal fibula's mobility by comparing one direction to the other, and wait for a subtle yielding or softening while applying static pressure in the stiffer direction.

Key points: Fibular Head Technique

Indications include:
- Type II dorsiflexion restriction.

Purpose
- Restore mobility and adaptability of distal fibula/tibia joint.

Instructions
- Sink into the fissure between tibia and fibula. Use gentle but firm pressure to encourage a slight widening of this fissure with dorsiflexion.

Movements
- Passive anterior and posterior glide of the fibula on the tibia.

Cautions
- Avoid painful pressure on the common peroneal nerve, just posterior to proximal fibular head.

More fibula facts

Here is some interesting trivia about the non-trivial fibula:

- There are seven named muscles that pull downwards or distally on the fibula (extensor hallucis and digitorum longii; peroneus longus, brevis, and tertius; tibialis posterior; and soleus), but only one (biceps femoris) that pulls upwards or proximally, leading some anatomists to speculate that the fibula is more often displaced inferiorly. However, the interosseous membrane of the leg (Figure 6.5) strongly resists this imbalanced downward pull on the fibula through its obliquely angled fibers, which are oriented to stabilize the fibula against the downward pull of the numerous leg muscles.

- The middle part of the fibula is sometimes used for bone graft reconstruction of the mandible. When "harvested" for this purpose, both of the fibula's ends are carefully left in place: the distal end, because of its special role in forming the ankle mortise; and the proximal

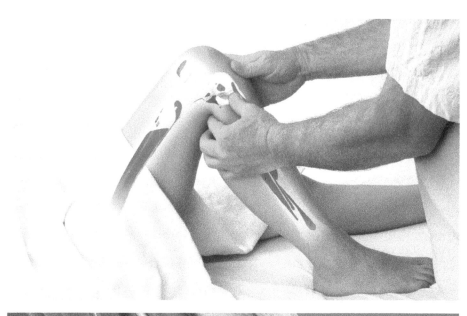

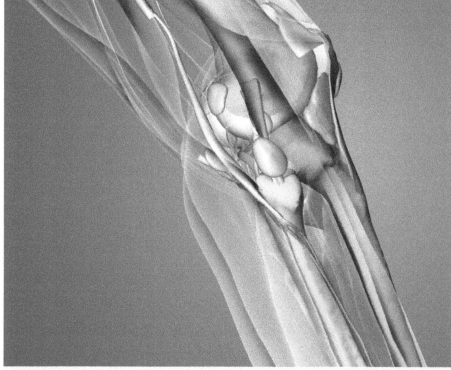

Figures 6.9/6.10

The Fibular Head Technique. Check for and release anterior/posterior mobility. Avoid pressure on the common peroneal nerve (yellow, Figure 6.9) where it lies posterior to the fibular head. (The fibula is colored green; the knee's many bursa are shown in blue).

end, because of its close association with the peroneal nerve.

- Since the fibula does not articulate with the femur, it is more functionally related to the ankle than the knee (at least in humans). Some animals' fibulas do not articulate with either foot bones or femurs, making their fibulae free at both ends. In horses, the tibia and fibula form a single joined bone.

As with any single body part, work the fibula as part of a bigger picture. For example, it is a good idea to prepare for the techniques outlined in this chapter by addressing any restrictions related to a tight gastrocnemius or soleus (Chapter 4), which will be a logical compliment to the work described in this chapter. Ankle pronation/supination, hip/knee/ankle alignment, as well as hip and femur rotation (Chapter 10, *Hip Mobility*), are all additional aspects to consider and address as part of your overall work with ankle and lower leg issues.

References

[1] American Academy of Orthopaedic Surgeons. *AOSSM Sports Tips: Ankle Sprains: How To Speed Your Recovery.* http://www.sportsmed.org/uploadedFiles/Content/Patient/Sports_Tips/ST%20Ankle%20Sprains%2008.pdf [Accessed 11/2013]

[2] American Academy of Orthopaedic Surgeons. Sprains and Strains: *What's the Difference?* http://orthoinfo.aaos.org/topic.cfm?topic=A00111 [Accessed 11/2013]

[3] Margo, K.L. (2008) Review: many adults still have pain and subjective instability at 1 year after acute lateral ankle sprain. *Evid Based Med.* 13(6). p. 187.

[4] Hartzell, D. and Shimmel, M. (2006) *Don't Ice that Ankle Sprain!* Jump Stretch, Inc.

[5] Kaminski, W.T. et al. (2013) National Athletic Trainers' Association Position Statement: Conservative Management and Prevention of Ankle Sprains in Athletes. *Journal of Athletic Training.* 48(4) p. 528–545.

[6] Kaminski (2013) (ibid)

[7] Kapandji, I.A. (1987) *Physiology of the Joints.* Vol. II, 5th ed. Philadelphia: Elsevier, p. 164.

[8] Kapandji (1987) (ibid)

[9] Bozkurt, M. et al. (2008) Axial rotation and mediolateral translation of the fibula during passive plantar flexion. *Foot Ankle Int.* 29(5) p. 502–7 PMID 18510904

[10] Beumer, A. et al. (2003) Kinematics of the distal tibiofibular syndesmosis: radiostereometry in 11 normal ankles. *Acta Orthop Scand*. 74 (3). p. 337–343

[11] Kapandji (1987) (ibid)

[12] Calhoun, J.H., Li, F., Ledbetter, B.R. et al. (1994) A comprehensive study of pressure distribution in the ankle joint with inversion and eversion. *Foot Ankle Int*. 15(3) p. 125–133.

[13] Rüedi, T.P. et al. (2007) *AO Principles of Fracture Management*. AO Foundation Publishing.

[14] Vicenzino, B. et al. (2007) Mulligan's mobilization-with-movement, positional faults and pain relief: current concepts from a critical review of literature. Man Ther. May; 12(2) p. 98–108.

Picture Credits

Study Guide

Ankle injuries and the Fibula

1   The Distal Tibiofibular Joint Technique encourages:
a   more side-to-side adaptability between the fibula and tibia
b   more firmness in the distal tibiofibular joint
c   a narrowing of the ankle mortise
d   more anterior/posterior shear of the ankle mortise

2   The study referred to in the text found that the only consistent risk factor for ankle injury is:
a   hyper-flexible ankles
b   inflexible ankles
c   a previous ankle sprain
d   high level of physical activity

3   According to the text, which of these is most commonly damaged in ankle injuries?
a   bones
b   fascia
c   bursa
d   nerves

4   According to the author, pressure on the fibula in which direction(s) can often provide relief from an inversion ankle sprain:
a   anteriorly and superiorly
b   posteriorly and superiorly
c   anteriorly and inferiorly
d   posteriorly and inferiorly

5   According to the text, the Distal Tibiofibular Joint Technique is used primarily when we find:
a   tight calf muscles
b   limited dorsiflexion of the foot
c   limited plantarflexion of the foot
d   supination of the foot

For Answer Keys, visit www.Advanced-Trainings.com/v1key/

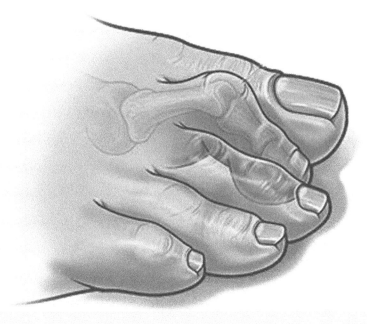

Figure 7.1

A hammertoe condition can involve soft tissue contracture in the toe, foot, and/or leg. Typically, a flexion fixation of the toe puts its end in contact with the ground, causing both pain and loss of foot function, which has far-reaching effects in the rest of the body.

My grandfather loved hunting quail while walking the fields and thickets of his native western Oklahoma prairie. At some point toward the end of his life, he switched from walking to driving, hanging his shotgun out the window of his old sedan, slowly cruising the back roads, still looking for quail. "It's my hammertoes," he'd say. "Just can't walk around like I used to."

A hammertoe is bent downwards (Figure 7.1), resulting in painful pressure either on the end of the toe or on its upper side, where it rubs or contacts the shoe. Common causes and risk factors include:

- Wearing narrow or tight-fitting shoes
- Imbalanced muscle strength, tonus, or flexibility in the foot or leg
- Direct trauma or injury to the structures involved
- Genetic influences, such as Morton's toe (the second toe being longer than the great toe making it more likely to be buckled by the end of the shoe
- Neuromuscular diseases (for example, multiple sclerosis, Charcot-Marie-Tooth disease, cerebral palsy), inflammatory diseases (for example, rheumatoid arthritis, psoriasis), and from the nerve damage that sometimes accompanies diabetes.

The second toe is most often affected (Figure 7.1), though hammertoe can be found in any of the toes. In a "true" hammertoe, the joint at the base of the toe (the metatarsal phalangeal joint, or MTPJ) and the next joint (the proximal interphangeal joint, or PIPJ) are fixed in a bent position. Variations include mallet toe (when the contracture occurs primarily at the most distal phalangeal joint, or DIPJ); claw toe (flexure at all three toe joints); crossover toe; and clinodactyly (congenitally curly toes). Our discussion will focus on hammertoes, but the principles and techniques discussed here can be adapted to address these other conditions as well.

Although the condition is seen in all ages (even at birth), the incidence of hammertoe increases with maturity, eventually affecting about one in ten people over the age of 60. Hammertoes are about five times more likely to occur in females than males (perhaps because women tend to wear tighter shoes than men – studies claim that nine out of ten women wear shoes that are too small) (1). There are racial differences as well; hammertoes occur about three times more frequently in African Americans under the age of 60 years than in whites of the same age (though there is much less racial difference observed in people over 60 years) (2).

Non-surgical care of hammertoe involves using more spacious shoes; padding points of contact; using special spacers, braces, or splints; physical therapy; and exercises (such as using just the toes to gather and ungather a towel on a hard floor).

Whatever the root cause or factors involved, the result is that with hammertoes, the soft tissues are too short to allow for the natural alignment of the toe bones. Surgeons address this problem by using one or more of the following methods:

1. Lengthening the contracted connective tissue by cutting toe tendons, capsules, or ligaments
2. Shortening bones to fit the contracted tissues by removing articular heads or other parts
3. In advanced cases, arthrodesis (fusion) of the bent joints via wires or other means is used in combination with the two methods described above.

Although some surgeons consider hammertoe surgery an "easy" surgery to perform (it is often the first surgery new surgeons are allowed to do) (3) complications do occur, and these most commonly include pain and discomfort related to

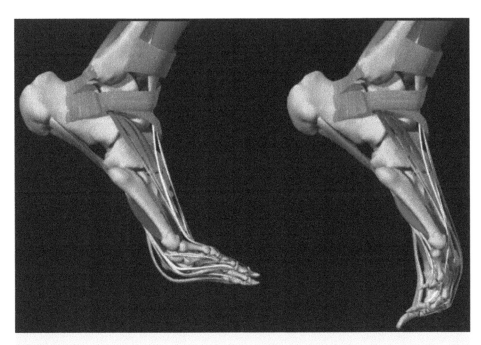

Figure 7.2

In normal movement, toe flexors and extensors take turns contracting and lengthening.

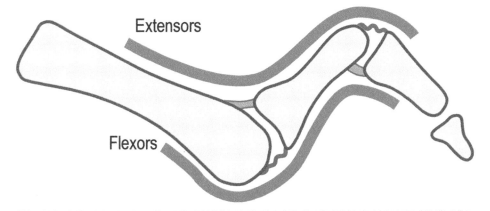

Figure 7.3

In hammertoes both flexors and extensors remain contracted simultaneously, buckling the toe. Over time, the ligaments and joint capsules can shorten, further fixing the joint.

the loss of movement in the toe, especially when joints have been excised or fused.

As manual therapists, there are many ways we can effectively release the shortened soft tissues involved in hammertoes and its related conditions. Sometimes this is corrective, reversing the curling of the toes, and other times it is palliative, meaning that it helps relieve the associated pain and other symptoms. It also is reasonable to imagine that soft tissue lengthening could, at least in some cases, delay or prevent hammertoe surgery, thus averting the resulting loss of mobility that patients often experience after corrective surgery.

Ida Rolf (the originator of Rolfing structural integration) said, "In a balanced body, when flexors flex, extensors extend" (Figure 7.2). Nowhere is this more obvious than in the toes. When toe flexors contract without reciprocal lengthening of the extensors, the toes are pulled short from both above and below. Since the toes cannot collapse like a telescope, nor is it easy for them to bend sideways (as the great toe does in hallux valgus or bunions), the middle toes shorten by buckling into a hammer (Figure 7.3), mallet, or claw shape, depending on the shape of the joint involved, as well as on the structures responsible for the pulling.

Locally, a hammertoe condition or other flexion fixation of the toe puts its end in contact with the ground, causing pain at the point of weight bearing and, often, on the upper (dorsal) surface of the toe where it contacts the shoe. In addition to pain, the lack of extension at the toe or toes causes a loss of whole-foot function.

Small things can have very big effects. Toes are a good example of this: when they are painful or do not bend properly, as in a hammertoe condition, they will make standing unbearable, throw off the stride, affect balance, and cause other troublesome compensations throughout the body.

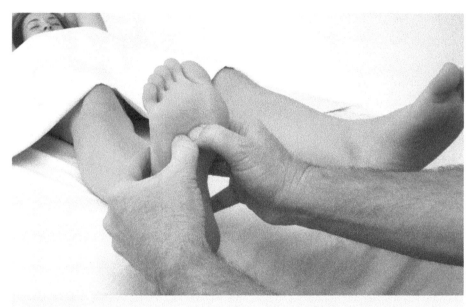

Figure 7.4

Use active or passive client movement to lengthen contracted toe flexors in the Flexor Digitorum Brevis technique.

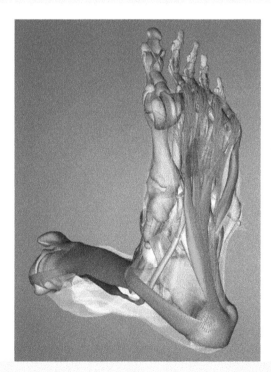

Figure 7.5

The short toe flexors (green). The long toe flexors (red) are also visible (and will be discussed in the Flexor Digitorum Longus Technique).

Functionally, the toes affect whole-body balance and movement. Structurally, hammertoes are not just a toe issue. Hammertoes can involve shortened and inelastic soft tissues in the toe itself, in the foot (via the flexor and extensor digitorum brevi), and/or in the leg, where the flexor and extensor digitorum longi can be especially strong contributors to fixing the toe in a flexed position. We will begin our work by addressing the foot and toes themselves, and then we will move on to the lower leg.

Flexor Digitorum Brevis Technique

When contracted, the short toe flexors in the sole of the foot (Figure 7.5) contribute to hammertoes by curling the PIPJ and DIPJ (the two distal joints of the toe). The flexors are found just deep to the plantar fascia, in the most superficial muscle layer at the bottom of the foot.

Before attempting to work with this muscle layer, begin by warming up the superficial and plantar fascias of the sole. These tissues can also contribute to toe flexure. Use any broad, superficial technique for this preparatory work (one example is the Plantar Fascia Technique, described in Chapter 4, *Type 1 Ankle Restrictions And Plantar Fasciitis*) Avoid using oil or cream, at least at this point, since reducing friction makes it more difficult to work with the sole's distinct tissue layers. Instead, slow down and let the tissues melt.

Once you have prepared the superficial and plantar fascias, use the tips of your curled thumbs to anchor the short, strong flexors in a heel-ward direction, as your client lifts his or her toes in active toe extension (Figure 7.4). You can also use passive toe extension, gently stretching the toes into extension with your free hand. This combination of anchoring into the short flexors and adding movement is very effective in lengthening contracted or shortened lines of strain in the underside of the foot. Be thorough, working

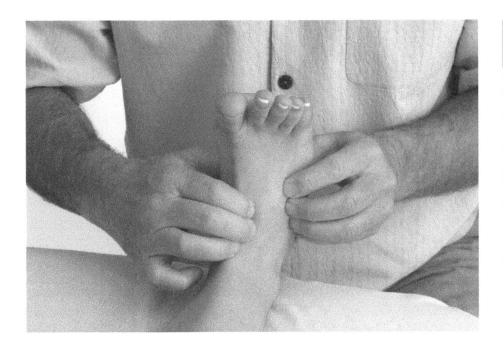

See video of the Extensor Digitorum Brevis Technique at http://advanced-trainings.com/v/la08.html

Key points: Flexor Digitorum Brevis (FDB) Technique

Indications include:
- Hammertoe, mallet toe, claw toe; pes cavus.
- Cramping of the sole of the foot.
- Limited toe flexion.

Purpose
- Restore lost elasticity and span of short toe flexors, tendons, tendon sheathes, and joint capsules.

Instructions
- After preparation work with plantar fascia and sole of the foot, anchor plantar-side tissues distally (towards heel) with curled thumbs. Use toe extension to lengthen tissues under your thumb tips.

Movements
- Active and passive toe extension.

Figures 7.6/7.7

The Extensor Digitorum Brevis Technique. By anchoring into the short toe extensors on the top of the foot, you may use active or passive toe flexion to lengthen the short toe extensors.

the entire sole, from the toes to the origin of the flexors on the anterior calcaneus.

Extensor Digitorum Brevis Technique

The extensor digitorum brevis (EDB) (Figure 7.8) is the only muscle (along with its hallucis head) on the dorsal surface of the foot. Functionally, it complements the short toe flexors by pulling the MTPJ (the joint at the base of the toe) into extension or dorsiflexion. When the EDB and its fasciae are short and inelastic, this up-bent dorsiflexion becomes the resting position of the toe joint. Use your fingertips (Figures 7.6 and 7.7) to release any contracted tissue here, this time using toe curling or flexion as active or passive client movements. Isolate each toe in turn, feeling for the specific head of the brevis involved in that toe's extension.

Toe tendons, capsules and sheaths

It will be important to spend some time working slowly and deeply around the joints of the toes

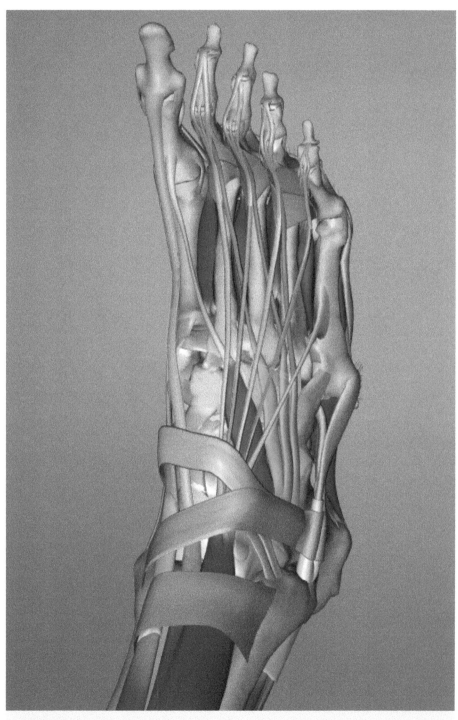

Figure 7.8
The extensor digitorum brevis (green).

Key points: Extensor Digitorum Brevis (EDB) Technique

Indications include:
- Hammertoe, mallet toe, claw toe.
- Limited toe flexion.

Purpose
- Restore lost elasticity and span of short toe extensors, tendons, tendon sheaths, and joint capsules.

Instructions
- Use fingertips to anchor dorsal foot tissues in a proximal direction. Use toe flexion to lengthen tissues under your fingertips.

Movements
- Active and passive toe extension.

---

themselves. Both the extensors (dorsally) and the flexors (on the plantar surface) merge with their longer counterparts (the flexor and extensor digitorum longus) into tendinous hoods within the toe (Figure 7.9). In a hammertoe pattern, these fibrous sheaths become contracted on the concave sides of the joint (in the crease of the bent toe; Figure 7.3).

The joint capsules, in addition to the toes' collateral ligaments, are also involved in maintaining a bent joint. The capsules wrap around all three toe joints, and are largest and strongest at the MTPJ, lying between the base of the toes. These ligaments and other structures between the long metatarsals of the foot, such as the adductors and lumbricals, will need to be gently lengthened before normal alignment is possible. As with our other techniques, use active and passive client movement along with your direct pressure to lengthen these shortened tissues.

If your client has already had hammertoe surgery but is still in pain, working the ligaments and tissues of the toes can often help reduce pain

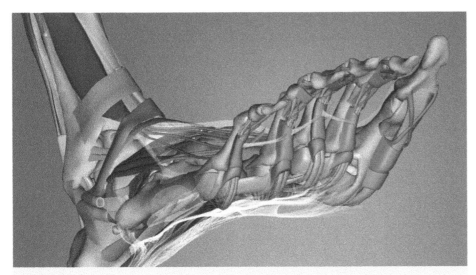

Figure 7.9

The flexor tendon sheaths (orange) are some of the fibrous connective tissue structures that surround the toe joints. They can contribute to toe joint fixation. Work these structures in detail, combining pressure with active and passive movement.

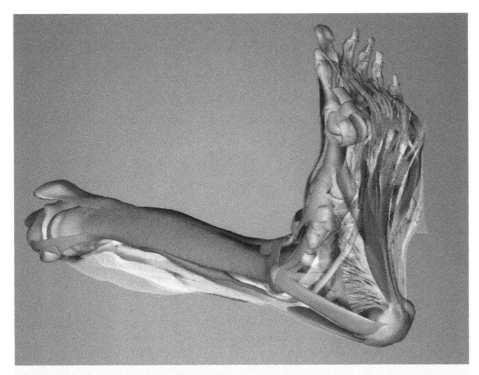

Figure 7.10

The extensor (red) and flexor (green) digitorum longus (red, anterior tibia) originate in the lower leg. Also pictured are the flexor digitorum brevis and minimus (red, within foot).

once the surgery has healed (after at least six to eight weeks).

Although the toes and their ligaments are sensitive, ticklish, or painful on many people, if you take your time and stay in close communication with your client, the sensation will be well tolerated. The normalization of hypersensitive areas can itself be very therapeutic. Combined with the tissue changes from your work, it will yield gratifying changes in flexibility and pain reduction.

At this point, you have worked the short toe flexors and extensors, as well as the sheaths, capsules, and ligaments of the toe joints themselves. Although there is more to do, and even though you may need repeated visits to see a visible change in your clients' toes' resting position, in many cases, your client will already notice greater toe flexibility and comfort.

Working the lower leg

So far, we have described a number of ways that you can work with the short toe flexors and extensors, as well as with the ligaments and tissues of the toes themselves. When shortened, these muscles and their associated tendons and fasciae are the main structures within the foot that contribute to hammertoe conditions; however, the foot structures are just part of the picture.

Flexor Digitorum Longus Technique

While working with the shorted structures within the foot is an essential part of addressing hammertoe patterns, the long toe flexors and extensors (Figure 7.10) exert even more contractile forces than their shorter brevi cousins. Originating in the lower leg, the long flexors and extensors cross the ankle and attach to the most distal bones of the toes, powerfully assisting in balance, stride push-off, jumping, toe pointing, and so on. As with their shorter brevi

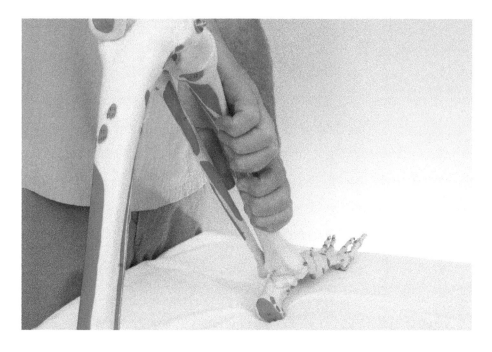

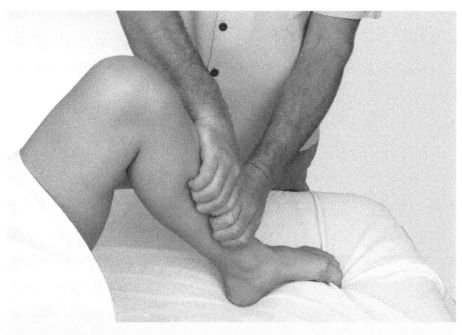

Figures 7.11/7.12

Flexor Digitorum Longus Technique. The long toe flexors lie on the posterior side of the tibia. This is a sensitive area and easily bruised, so use gentle pressure and active toe flexion (curling), rather than sliding or moving your fingers.

counterparts within the foot, when both the long flexors and extensors are shortened, they buckle the DIPJ and PIPJ (the joints of the toe itself), as well as the MTPJ at the base of the toe.

Even though they affect the toe joints, the main part of the long toe flexors and extensors are in the lower leg. We will address these components by utilizing the Golgi tendon organ reflex. When stimulated with a combination of pressure and active movement, the Golgi tendon organs (which are often concentrated near a tendon's attachments to the periosteum) signal the motor units' alpha motor neurons (via synapses in the spinal cord) to lower that muscle's firing rate. With minimal effort on the part of the practitioner, working a muscle's attachments and stimulating this Golgi response results in a reduction in local hypertonus, and enhances finer global movement coordination (4).

The proximal attachments of the flexor digitorum longus can be accessed on the medial side of the lower leg, midway between ankle and knee, on the posterior aspect of the tibia (Figures 7.11, 7.12, and 7.13). To stimulate a Golgi response here, wrap your hands around the shin and feel into the structures just behind the tibia with your fingers. This is a sensitive area, so proceed slowly. By asking your client to flex (curl) his or her toes, you will be able to locate the precise attachments of the flexor digitorum longus on the posterior side of the tibia. Rather than sliding or scrubbing, use firm but gentle static pressure here, as your client continues to actively curl and uncurl the toes. Asking your client to "gather up the sheet with your toes" is an effective cue. Feel for a release and softening of the tissues under your touch, and also feel for a shift in the initiation of your client's movement. Once the Golgi response has engaged, movements will initiate more gradually and smoothly, and with finer control; in other words, with less of an initial jerk or all-or-nothing contraction.

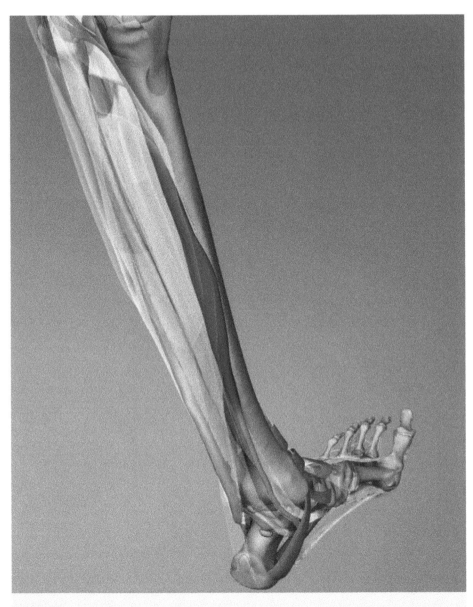

Figure 7.13
The flexor digitorum longus (red).

Repeat this slow, steady release in several places along the mid-section of the tibia where the flexor attaches, right up next to the bone, wherever you feel muscle contraction with toe flexion. Then, finish your work here with longer or gliding strokes to ease out of this sensitive area.

Working the long flexors in this way will addresses toe curling (flexion) fixations. We will complement this with work on the long toe extensors to address the upward bending (extension) of the MTPJ.

> **Key points:** Flexor Digitorum Longus (FDL) Technique
>
> **Indications include:**
> - Hammertoe, mallet toe, claw toe; pes cavus.
> - Limited toe extension.
> - Type 1 ankle dorsiflexion restrictions.
>
> **Purpose**
> - Reduce resting tone and restore lost elasticity of the long toe extensors via a Golgi tendon organ response.
>
> **Instructions**
> - Use sensitive static pressure on FDL attachments on medial side of posterior tibia. Use active toe and ankle motions to refine your placement, and to evoke a Golgi tendon organ response. Feel for smoother, slower initiation of movement, and softening of tissues under your fingertips.
>
> **Movements**
> - Active toe flexion and extension; active ankle dorsiflexion and plantarflexion.

Extensor Digitorum Longus Technique

The extensor digitorum longus (EDL) attaches to the medial surface of fibula, and runs along the proximal three-fourths of that bone's length. It also attaches to the intermuscular septa and

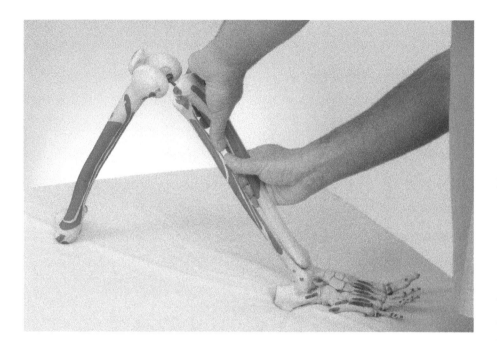

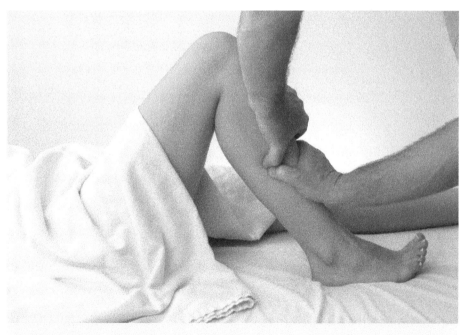

Figures 7.14/7.15

Extensor Digitorum Longus Technique. The long toe extensors attach to the fibula, and to the interosseous membrane of the leg in the space between the tibia and fibula. Use active toe extension in combination with static pressure on these structures' proximal attachments.

the interosseous membrane of the leg, which span the space between the fibula and tibia.

To work the long toe extensor attachments, use the same around-the-shin grip that you used for the flexor digitorum longus techniques, but this time, your thumbs will do the work (Figures 7.14 and 7.15). Find the front of the fibula by sinking in just anterior to the long, ropy peroneals on the lateral side of the leg. Take care of your thumbs by avoiding hyperextension – maintain slight flexion in each of your thumbs' joints. The extensor attachments can be tricky to find – the tissue here is dense, compact, and undifferentiated on many people. Sometimes, using a broader, more superficial technique to prepare the front of the leg first can help make the extensor attachments more accessible. One such technique may include the Tibialis Anterior Technique, which is described in Chapter 5.

Once you come in contact with the muscle attachments on the bone itself, focus on the fibula's anteromedial aspect. As with the previous technique, use static pressure together with active toe movements to help locate and release the attachments. This time, use toe extension (lifting the toes). For the release phase, a cue could be "push the sheet out from under your foot by uncurling your toes;" in other words, this is the reverse of the movements used for the long flexors. As with that technique, feel for tissue release, together with a shift towards slower, smoother initiation of movement, as these are indicators of a Golgi response. Once you feel these things, move to different areas of the fibula, as well as into the space between the tibia and fibula to work the attachments on the interosseous membrane.

The Tibialis Anterior Technique mentioned above (or a similar broad technique) can also serve as a finishing move to smooth out the areas worked, especially if your focused pressure left edematous

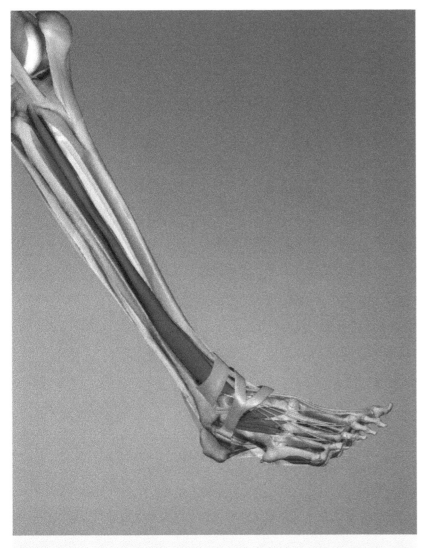

Figure 7.16

The extensor digitorum longus and brevis (red).

Indications include:
- Hammertoe, mallet toe, claw toe.
- Limited toe flexion, especially when further reduced by ankle plantarflexion.

Purpose
- Reduce resting tone and restore lost elasticity of the long toe flexors via a Golgi tendon organ response.

Instructions
- After preparing the overlying tissues, use sensitive static pressure on EDL attachments on medial side of anterior fibula. Use active toe and ankle motions to refine your placement, and to evoke a Golgi tendon organ response. Feel for smoother, slower initiation of movement, and softening of tissues under your fingertips.

Movements
- Active toe flexion and extension; active ankle dorsiflexion and plantarflexion.

depressions in the front of the leg (not uncommon, and typically not a cause for concern).

What about bunions?

Hallux valgus or bunions (Figure 7.17) often accompanies hammertoes. Bunions are thought to sometimes cause hammertoes through the lateral crowding that the great toe exerts on the smaller toes. However, it also seems plausible that the same soft tissue imbalances that contribute to hammertoe contracture could cause halux valgus. While the smaller toes are stabilized by their neighbors and buckle more easily in the sagittal plane (flexion/extension), the great toe buckles easiest in the transverse plane (abduction/adduction). In other words, when the flexors and extensors are both short,

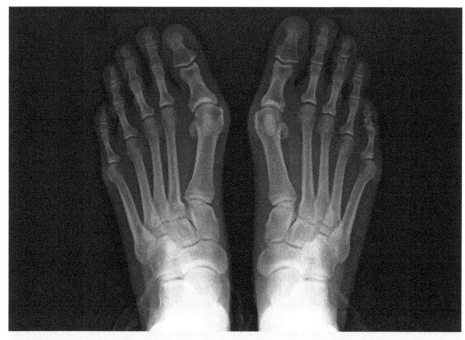

Figure 7.17

Hallux valgus or bunions can accompany hammertoes. You can sometimes ease bunion rigidity and pain by working the flexor and extensor hallucis, both longus and brevis, in ways similar to those described here for the toe flexors and extensors.

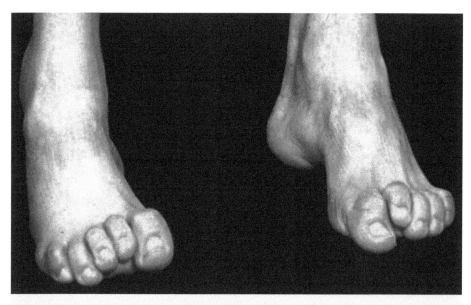

Figure 7.18

Hammertoes or bunions often accompany other conditions involving connective tissue contracture, such as pes talipes (also known as pes cavus or clubfoot).

the smaller toes buckle into a hammertoe position, and the big toe buckles into a bunion.

Hallux valgus can also be related to such factors as external femur rotation, tight-fitting shoes, genetic contributors, and other influences. Whatever their cause, I have observed that working the flexor and extensor hallucis in ways similar to what has been described here can help relieve the soft-tissue contributions to bunion discomfort and rigidity.

Hammertoes and bunions do not exist in isolation – their fixity and tissue shortness reflect patterns that occur elsewhere in the body. For instance, hammertoes are often present when the foot shows a high degree of overall connective tissue contracture, such as high fixed arches or, in extreme examples, talipes or pes cavus (clubfoot) (Figure 7.18). Hammertoe contraction is not limited to the toe muscles – in my experience, hammertoes can be accompanied by tighter hamstrings, spinal erectors, and cervical muscles; exaggerated spinal curves; and other patterns of connective tissue shortness throughout the body. Similarly, restricted toe motion will have whole-body effects, subsequently shortening a person's stride, increasing his or her leg rotation and head-bob, impairing his or her balance, changing the knee and hip dynamics, and so on.

Can joints change?

The curl of hammertoes can be more or less mobile, ranging from fairly flexible and springy, to quite fixed and rigid. Although hammertoes usually start as soft tissue contractures, over time the stress of the bent position, lack of movement, and pressure from shoe contact can degrade the articular surfaces of the toe joints, causing articular rigidity and additional pain. The more rigid the toe joints are, the more likely it is that there are bony or articular changes.

This is not a reason to give up working with them. I mentioned that my grandfather complained about his toe pain. By his nineties, when I began working with his hammertoes, his elderly joints were quite rigid and probably had a high degree of joint degeneration, but our work yielded very worthwhile results nonetheless – he had significantly improved toe and foot mobility, and this helped him to become increasingly steadier on his feet and easier in his stance.

Bones and joints themselves can change for the better; when normal tissue tone and movement is restored, joints can and do heal. This notwithstanding, there are clearly times when surgical interventions may be the best available remedy. For clients who have had toe surgery, once the tissues have healed, these techniques are very effective in helping reestablish a more normal range of motion and function.

Given that hammertoes sometimes result from disease, neuropathology, or other issues, we obviously will not be able to reverse every case of hammertoes. But even in these cases, your skillful and thorough soft-tissue work will help relieve your client's pain and help prevent further loss of movement and resultant degeneration.

If there are articular rigidities – irrespective of their cause – it simply means you and your client need to be more modest in your expectations for a quick fix. Be patient and persistent, use your client's active movements, and be sure to notice the small, incremental improvements as they occur.

References

[1] *Hammertoes/Claw Toes*. (20 Sep 2011) http://www.healthcommunities. com/hammertoesclaw-toes/hammertoe-remedies.shtml. [Accessed Jan 2014]

[2] Watson, A. (2009) Hammertoe Deformity. eMedicine. Ed. Stephens, H.M. 10 Mar. *Medscape*. 23 Jun.

[3] Fishco, W. (2009) Emerging Concepts in Hammertoe Surgery. *Podiatry Today*. 22(9). p. 34.

[4] Schleip, R. (2003) Fascial Plasticity – A New Neurobiological Explanation, Part I. *Journal of Bodywork and Movement Therapies* 7, no. 1. p. 14.

Picture credits

Figure 7.1 courtesy Healthwise, used by permission.

Figure 7.3 courtesy Advanced-Trainings.com (after Cailliet), used by permission.

Figures 7.2, 7.4, 7.5 and 7.8 and 7.9, 7.10, 7.13, 7.16 and 7.18 courtesy Primal Pictures, used by permission.

Figures 7.6, 7.7, 7.11, 7.12, 7.14 and 7.15 courtesy Advanced-Trainings.com, used by permission.

Figure 7.17 copyright Michael Nebel, used under CC BY-SA license.

Study Guide

Hammertoes

1 **Where are the flexor digitorum brevi found?**

a top of the foot
b posterior lateral leg
c bottom of the foot
d medial tibia

2 **According to Ida Rolf, in a balanced body when the flexors flex, the extensors:**

a shorten
b extend
c separate
d hurt

3 **As described in the text, what client movement is used in the Flexor Digitorum Brevis Technique?**

a ankle inversion
b toe flexion
c ankle plantarflexion
d toe extension

4 **The text states that the Golgi tendon organs are concentrated where:**

a in the belly of the muscle
b near muscle attachments
c inside the joint capsule
d in ligaments

5 **As stated in the text, the practitioner's hands in the Flexor Digitorum Longus Technique:**

a slide along the tibia
b hold static pressure on the lateral posterior fibula
c hold static pressure on the medial posterior tibia
d slide along the lateral posterior fibula

For Answer Keys, visit www.Advanced-Trainings.com/v1key/

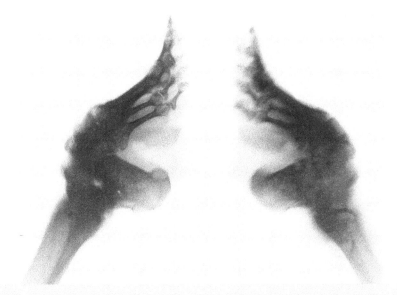

Figure 8.1
An X-ray of bound feet.

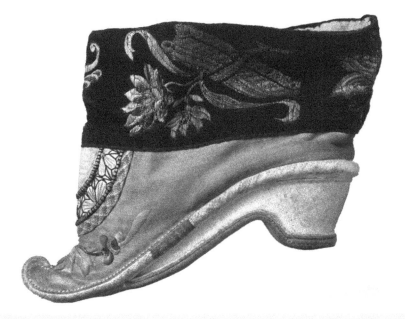

Figure 8.2
A miniature shoe for a bound foot, China, 18th century. Images are sized to approximately the same scale, as the shoe was worn only on the big toe.

Michelangelo said, "What spirit is so empty and blind, that it cannot recognize that the foot is more noble than the shoe?" Some 500 years later, we are still squeezing our feet into shoes; shoes that, in the name of beauty, are often too small.

However, compressed feet are rarely happy feet. As an extreme example, consider foot binding, which was practiced in some parts of China until modern times, despite being outlawed in 1912 and again in 1949. In the name of beauty, the foot bones were broken and distorted to allow the wearing of a miniature shoe (Figures 8.1 and 8.2). Women with bound feet suffered pain and lifelong disabilities (1).

The space between the foot bones is as important as the bones themselves. Without enough space, the feet lose their supple mobility, which is needed for adapting to the constantly changing angles, forces, and surfaces that standing, walking, and running entail. When the feet are not able to make the ultra-fine adjustments that provide stability, structures elsewhere in the body must compensate. Muscles grip; connective tissues harden, tighten, and eventually solidify to make up for the foot's loss of adaptable function.

Try this: walk barefoot around the room, but stiffen one of your big toe joints – do not allow it to move. This will change the way you walk; see if you can notice where else in your body you feel the effects of this toe restriction. If you had to walk like this for a long time, where would you need some hands-on work? Many will notice a change in their knee function, or they may find that they have stiffer hips, or back or neck discomfort. When the feet are not happy, the rest of the body is not happy.

Barefoot is how we're meant to walk and run, argued an influential 2004 paper in *Nature* that many see as the launch of the barefoot running

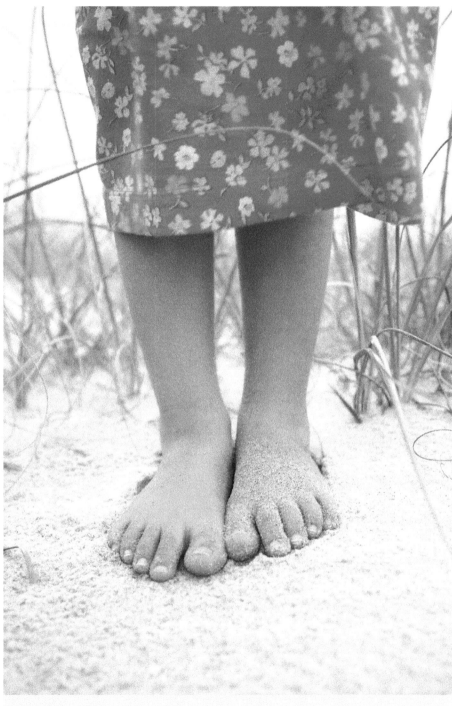

Figure 8.3
Research comparing shoe-users' feet with those of indigenous non-shoe users correlates shoe use with narrower feet, higher arches, and less-even weight distribution.

trend (2). Minimalist running quickly gained popularity with the publication of Christopher McDougall's 2009 bestseller *Born to Run*. About five years later, as this volume goes to press, barefoot running seems to be just as suddenly losing popularity, as reports of injuries mount (3). The evidence is mixed, however, and barefoot running still has both fervent adherents and crusading detractors. Although clearly not a panacea, and notwithstanding its faddish aspects (minimalist shoes, in spite of having less to them, often cost more), barefoot running spurred a thought-provoking debate into the definition of foot health. This debate offers ideas that we can adopt for our hands-on work with clients and patients. For example, advocates of barefoot running hold that our bodies do better when the feet are not over-cushioned or immobilized, as over-cushioning can reduce the proprioceptive signal that foot-strike provides.

I will describe two techniques in this chapter that can help anyone's feet regain a higher degree of natural mobility and adaptability, whether they run barefoot or not.

Are flat feet bad feet?

Looking at the issue of arch height, a quick overview of arch anatomy is in order. Skeletally, the foot bones function as sets of longitudinal rays, each comprised of a toe, its metatarsal, and an associated tarsal bone. These foot rays are further grouped into two structural divisions: the medial and lateral arches (Figure 8.3). The bones of the medial arch include the phalanges of toes one, two, and three; their metatarsals; plus the cuneiforms, navicular, and talus. The lateral arch is made up of toe rays four and five, which share the cuboid as their associated tarsal. The cuboid, in turn, articulates with the calcaneus via a unique locking joint, which adds stability. The connective tissues – muscles, tendons, ligaments, fascias, and joint capsules of the foot and

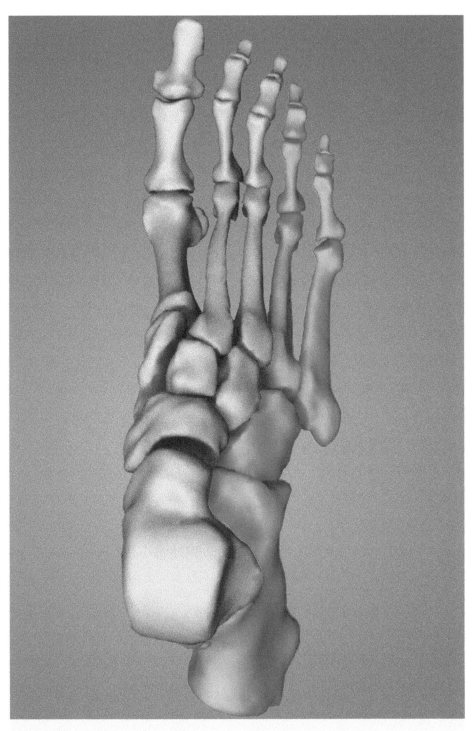

Figure 8.4

The skeletal divisions of the foot: the medial arch and the lateral arch (purple).

lower leg – contribute either spring or fixity to the arches, depending on the tissues' elasticity and resilience.

Conventionally, low arches or flat feet have been thought to be problematic, though some proponents of barefoot running question this assumption. While over-pronation (Figure 8.4) has clearly been linked to foot, ankle, and leg problems, the relationship of arch height to pronation and overall foot health is not as clear.

The generally accepted view links low arches with over-pronation of the calcaneus. Because the talus (part of the medial arch) rests on top of the calcaneus (which is part of the lateral arch), pronation or eversion of the calcaneus and lateral arch is conventionally thought to dump the talus medially, lowering the medial arch and giving rise to flat feet. However, there is credible research that contradicts this view, correlating pronation with higher arches, rather than lower ones (Figure 8.5) (4). Studies suggest that barefoot running can reduce over-pronation, even though it eschews the arch support that shoes are conventionally thought to provide (5). There is also ample evidence that shoe use increases foot narrowing and arch height. One study (comparing indigenous non-shoe wearers with developed-world habitual shoe-wearers) correlated shoe use with higher arches and narrowed feet, and showed less-even weight distribution in the sole when compared to non-shoe users (6). Other researchers question the reliability, relevance, and usefulness of arch height measurements in general (7).

Where does this leave us? Rather than assuming that a foot has problems based on its arch height (or lack thereof), we can take the pragmatic approach of assessing and releasing articular immobility and connective tissue restrictions wherever we find them, working toward the structural differentiation that brings resilience and adaptability. In addition to more balanced foot mobility, it is also important to include symptom improvement (less pain in the feet or elsewhere) and our clients' subjective experience (do the feet simply feel better?) as our indicators of success. Using these three factors as our goals – adaptability, symptom improvement, and subjective experience – is often more effective, and probably more universally relevant, than trying to produce changes in foot shape or arch height alone.

Transverse Arch Technique

We will begin our work by releasing any superficial or deep restrictions to the transverse arch's adaptability and to midfoot width. Shoes often squeeze the feet, challenging their ability to maintain their natural mediolateral adaptability. This squeezing has the effect of immobilizing the relationship between the medial and lateral arches, resulting in a transverse arch with less spring and recoil. This broad technique allows you to assess and release restrictions to mediolateral arch adaptability, and it is ideal preparation for our deeper work with the arches.

Facing the dorsal surface (top) of the foot, grasp the medial and lateral arches (Figure 8.6). Feel for the outer layers at first – the skin, and just underneath it, the various layers of enveloping fascias. These include the fascia dorsalis pedis (Figure 8.7), which wraps the foot and is continuous with the more fibrous extensor retinacula addressed in Chapter 6. Use a firm but sensitive grip. Once you feel these layers, use your fingertips on the sole of the foot as a fulcrum, as you roll (flex) your wrists apart to spread the tissue layers on top of the foot. This rolling and spreading accentuates the depth of the transverse arch, allowing you to feel and release any mobility restrictions that might be preventing arch adaptability.

Repeat this slow, firm rolling and spreading with successively deeper layers in turn, working in both distal and proximal positions, until you feel

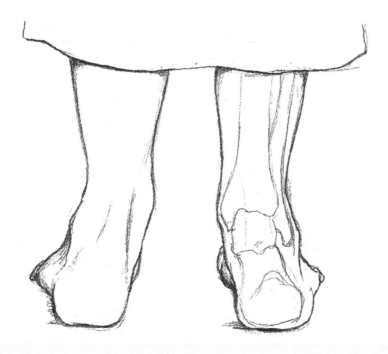

Figure 8.5

Over-pronation of the subtalar joint can cause problems, but some studies suggest it may be linked to high arches, rather than low arches as conventionally assumed.

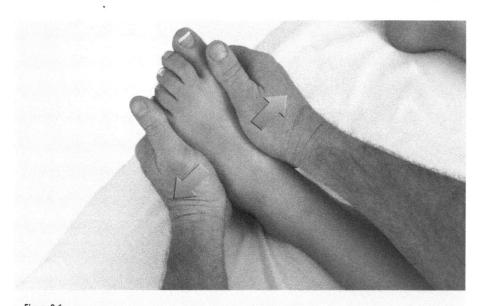

Figure 8.6

In the Transverse Arch Technique, work successively deeper layers of the foot with a spreading motion in order to assess and release mediolateral transverse arch mobility.

increased mobility of the tarsal and metatarsal bones in both the superficial layers and deep within the foot.

Arch Mobility Technique

The metatarsals are lined up side-by-side in the midfoot, much like sardines in a can. This side-by-side arrangement helps the metatarsals resist excessive lateral movement, while allowing them to spring up and down in the sagittal plane. This controlled dorsal/plantar mobility of the metatarsus allows the connective tissues of the foot (such as the tendons, plantar fascia, and spring ligaments) to absorb shock and store energy for release into the next step. When the metatarsals are fixed, undifferentiated, and immobile, the foot lacks both the spring and adaptability necessary for efficient and comfortable function.

Begin the Arch Mobility Technique by assessing the motion of the individual metatarsal bones. Using a firm grip, move two rays of the foot against each other in the sagittal plane (Figure 8.8). This does not involve squeezing

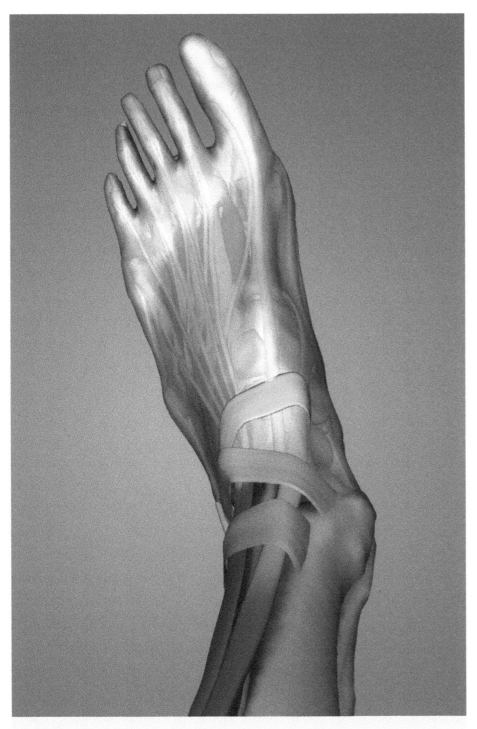

Figure 8.7

The fasciae of the foot include the fascia dorsalis pedis (grey), which is continuous with the extensor retinacula (tan).

Key points: Transverse Arch Technique

Indications include:
- Loss of transverse arch width, adaptability and flexibility.
- Pronation/supination imbalance.
- Morton's neuroma.

Purpose
- Assess and release restrictions to transverse arch adaptability and foot width.

Instructions
- Working each fascial layer from superficial to deep, spread and mediolaterally mobilize the bony rays of the foot, particularly across the foots dorsum (upper surface) in order to accentuate the transverse arch.

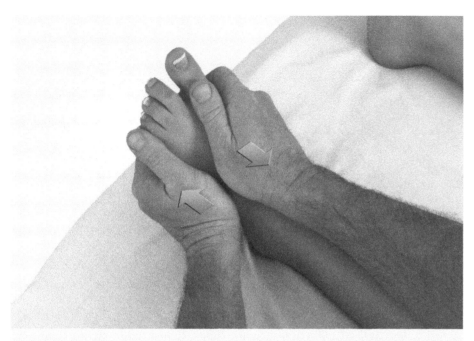

Figure 8.8

The Arch Mobility Technique. Dorsal/plantar mobility of the metatarsals allows for arch spring and foot adaptability. Use an up/down shearing motion, in both directions, to assess and release each metatarsal ray of the foot.

and releasing, nor does it include kneading the soft tissue of the foot. With a constant amount of grip pressure, isolate the up/down (dorsal/plantar) motion of each metatarsal bone in turn, moving it back and forth against its neighbor in a slow but full scrubbing motion.

Feel for mobility restrictions in either direction. When you find a direction that is less free, use the same full anterior/posterior motion to increase mobility. Make sure the distal ends of the metatarsal are mobile, as this will lay the groundwork for individual toe adaptability and range. Check and release the proximal ends of the metatarsals as well, along with each accompanying tarsal bone. Be thorough, scrubbing each pair of metatarsal rays against one another in turn.

Especially important is the division between the rays of toes three and four, since this is where the medial arch meets the lateral arch (Figure 8.3). This division extends proximally between the third cuneiform and the cuboid, and then between the talus and the calcaneus, and it is often the first intermetatarsal space to lose adaptability. When this functional cleavage line is not mobile, the arches become fixed in

Key points: Arch Mobility Technique

Indications include:
- Loss of dorsal/plantar tarsal and metatarsal mobility and flexibility.
- Pronation/supination imbalance.

Purpose
- Assess and release restrictions to foot bone mobility in the sagittal plane to restore arch mobility and resilience.

Instructions
- Using a firm grip, move each pair of adjacent foot rays against each other in the sagittal plane (anteroposteriorly), feeling for and releasing restrictions to free mobility.

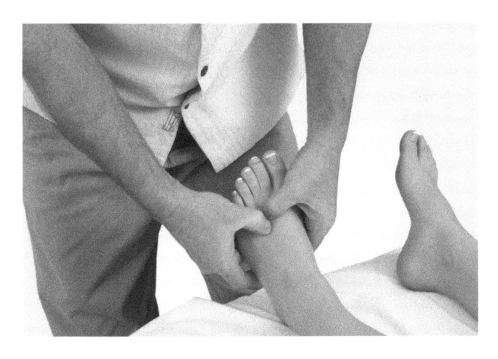

relation to one another, negatively affecting the pronation/supination balance, arch spring, and overall adaptability of the foot and ankle.

Intermetatarsal Technique

See video of the Intermetatarsal Technique at http://advanced-trainings.com/v/la04.html

It bears repeating: the spaces between the bones are just as important as the bones themselves. Without the differentiation that gives adaptability, strength turns to rigidity, both in the feet and in the rest of the body. The Intermetatarsal Technique is a straightforward way to regain lost lateral differentiation and adaptability in the forefoot.

Using your thumb and fingers, feel into the space between each metatarsal from above and below the foot. Allowing for your client's comfort level, use enough pressure to feel all the way through the foot, as if touching the thumb and fingers together between the bones (Figures 8.9 and 8.10). As always, avoid pressure that elicits sharp, electric, or other uncomfortable sensations, since there are sensitive nerves in the intermetatarsal spaces. Once your fingers and thumbs are in position, wait for the foot to yield. In the time it takes the tissues to respond, you can typically take two or three slow breaths of your own.

After you feel the initial release, you can facilitate a deeper and more sustainable response by asking your client for slow, focused, active movement. Have your client gradually flex and extend his or her toes, and then the ankle, as you maintain the space between the metatarsals with your fingers and thumb. There is almost no movement of your touch; any sliding that occurs results from your client's active movements. In addition to helping the tissues release, holding the bones apart as your client moves adds an element of movement reeducation, as your client's nervous system learns what it feels like to move the foot, while maintaining width across the foot. Repeat

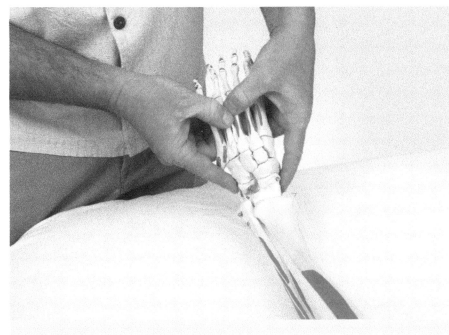

Figures 8.9/8.10

The Intermetatarsal Technique with a static touch, work between each pair of bones from both above and below, as if touching the fingers and thumb together through the foot. Once the tissue has responded, ask for slow toe and ankle movement.

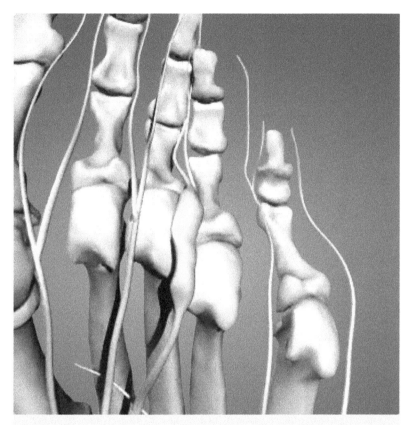

Figure 8.11
Morton's neuroma, a painful fibrotic enlargement of the nerve's connective tissue sheath, is one symptom associated with crowding of the metatarsals.

this cycle of a sustained, static-touch release, followed by active movement in several places along each metatarsal space, and then between all other pairs of foot rays, for both feet.

Morton's neuroma

In some people, the narrowing of the metatarsals can irritate and enlarge the perineurium (the outer connective tissue layer) of the intermetatarsal branches of the plantar nerve (Figure 8.11), causing foot pain or numbness. This condition, known as Morton's neuroma, occurs about 80–85 percent of the time between the third and fourth metatarsals, right where the medial arch meets the lateral arch (8). (The remaining 15–20 percent of cases occur between the second and third metatarsal, and are not thought to occur in other intermetatarsal spaces.) If your client complains of numbness or a sharp pain between the distal ends of the metatarsals, especially when standing or wearing shoes, work to separate and

Key points: Intermetatarsal Technique

Indications include:
- Loss of intermetatarsal space and adaptability.
- Morton's neuroma.

Purpose
- Reestablish foot width, arch differentiation, and adaptability.
- Neuromuscular movement reeducation and proprioceptive refinement.

Instructions
- Sensitively feel into the space between each metatarsal from above and below the foot. Wait in each space for sensation and tissue change. Add active movement to facilitate tissue change and nervous system response.

Movements
- Slow, small active toe flexion and extension; active ankle dorsiflexion and plantarflexion.

decompress the intermetatarsal spaces. As long as it is within your client's comfort range, gentle but deep work here can help ease the effects of midfoot narrowing and compression, as well as address the connective tissue fibrosity of the perineurium and its surrounding tissues. Use your client's active toe flexion and extension to glide the tissues under your fingertips; feel for an increase in bony mobility and openness of the intermetatarsal space. Your client may experience rapid relief, but do not be discouraged if it takes several sessions before the irritation subsides. Stubborn cases merit a change of footwear and/or evaluation by a specialist. Conventional non-surgical treatments include orthotics, orthopedic pads, or sclerosing injections to block nerve pain using controlled scarring. Your hands-on work can effectively support, augment, and complement each of these methods.

Just like people, not all feet are the same. Barefoot running is not for everyone, and what works for one client may need to be adapted or avoided for another. We will be most effective as practitioners if we bring the desired qualities of adaptability and flexibility to our own strategizing as well. After all, as psychiatrist Carl Jung said,

"The shoe that fits one person pinches another; there is no recipe for living that suits all cases."

References

[1] For more images and information about foot binding, see www.environmentalgraffiti.com/news-foot-binding.

[2] Bramble. D. and Lieberman, D.E. (2004) Endurance running and the evolution of Homo. *Nature*. Nov 18; 432(7015). p. 345–352.

[3] Germano, S. (2014) Barefoot' Running Heads Into the Sunset. *Wall Street Journal*. May 8, 2014.

[4] Boozer, et al. (2002) Investigation of the Relationship between Arch Height and Maximum Pronation Angle During Running. *Biomedical Sciences Instrumentation 38*. p. 203–207.

[5] A. Stacoff, et al. (1991) The Effects of Shoes on the Torsion and Rearfoot Motion in Running. *Medicine and Science in Sports and Exercise 23*. 4. p. 482–490.

[6] D'aout, K. et al. (2009) The Effects of Habitual Footwear Use: Foot Shape and Function in Native Barefoot Walkers. *Footwear Science 1*. p. 81–94.

[7] Menz, H. (1998) Alternative Techniques for the Clinical Assessment of Foot Pronation. *Journal of the American Podiatric Medical Association*. 88(3). p. 119–129.

[8] Wheeless, C. (2013) *Wheeless' Textbook of Orthopaedics*. http://www.wheelessonline.com/ortho/mortons_neuroma_interdigital_perineural_fibrosis. [Accessed January 2014]

Picture credits

Figures 8.1 and 8.2 in the public domain.

Figure 8.3 courtesy Primal Pictures, used by permission.

Figure 8.4 courtesy Léo Washburn, used by permission.

Figure 8.5 courtesy Thinkstock, used by permission.

Figures 8.6–8.10 courtesy Advanced-Trainings.com, used by permission.

Figure 8.11 courtesy Primal Pictures, used by permission.

Study Guide

The Shoe-Bound Arch

1 **In the opening paragraphs, what does the author say is just as important as the bones of the foot?**

a the connective tissues of the foot
b the space between the bones
c the ligaments of the foot
d the postural alignment of the foot

2 **According to the chapter, the rays of the foot are grouped into what two structural divisions?**

a the forefoot and hind foot
b the tarsals and metatarsals
c the medial and lateral arches
d the medial and transverse arches

3 **According to the text, which tarsal bone articulates with the calcaneus via a unique locking joint?**

a the navicular
b the cuboid
c the talus
d the sesamoid

4 **Which of these best describes the hand movement the practitioner uses in the Transverse Arch Technique?**

a an up and down movement
b sustained digital pressure
c rolling and spreading
d squeezing the space between the bones

5 **As described in the text, how does the practitioner assess metatarsal mobility in the Arch Mobility Technique?**

a by spreading the foot medio-laterally
b by longitudinally torsioning the foot
c by squeezing between the bones of the foot
d by using an up and down motion

For Answer Keys, visit www.Advanced-Trainings.com/v1key/

Hamstring Injuries

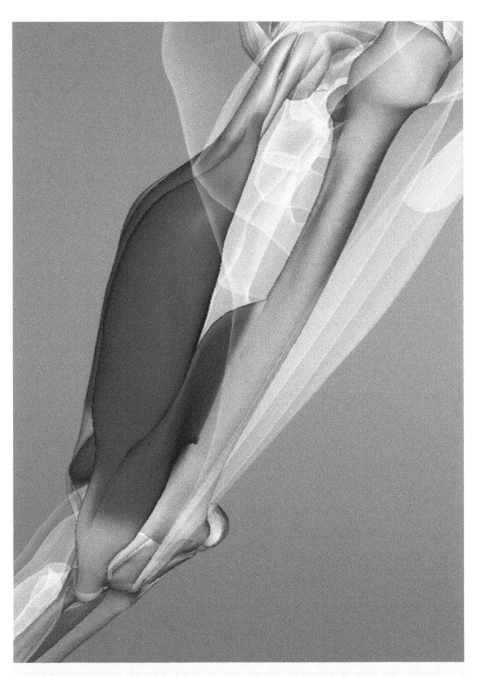

Figure 9.1

The hamstrings are powerful structures that are involved in running, striding, and jumping. The biceps femoris (the hamstring closest to the viewer in this image) is most commonly injured.

Which word first comes to mind when you hear *hamstrings*? If you said "tight," "sore," "pulled," or "injured," you have plenty of company – these are the words most frequently used with *hamstrings* in Google searches. It does not take a psychoanalyst to interpret those free-association results – many people associate hamstrings with pain, stiffness, and injury.

Hamstrings work hard. They are major stabilizers of the body's biggest segmental relationships, such as pelvic tilt, trunk angle, and hip position. They are also prime movers in some of the body's most powerful actions, such as running, stepping, jumping, and bending (Figure 9.1). As such, they are prone to straining or tearing injuries (Figure 9.2), most often as a result of sudden acceleration or of lunging motions, such as those common in running and ball sports.

The most common sites for hamstring injuries are:

1. At their musculotendinous junctions (usually mid-thigh, where the tendons blend with muscle fibers).
2. At the hamstrings' proximal end, at their tendinous insertions on the ischium.
3. The hamstrings are comprised of the semimembranosus, semitendinosus, and biceps femoris. The biceps femoris is the most lateral part of these muscles (Figure 9.1), and is the most frequently injured of this group.

Given that hamstring strains usually result from activity, they occur most often in active people, and active people sometimes have difficulty not being active. This might be why re-injury of partially recovered strains or tears is quite common. About one-third of recovering athletes re-injure their hamstrings, most often within the first 14 days after returning to play (1). Hamstring

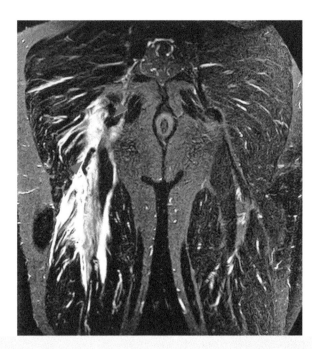

Figure 9.2

Coronal section MRI of a torn hamstring tendon (red arrows). Bleed-out into surrounding tissues is also visible.

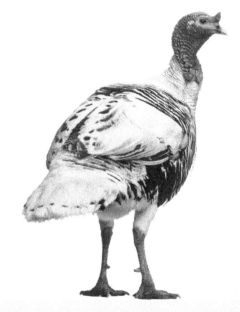

Figure 9.3

Turkeys develop bone-like structures within their hamstring tendons; they also spend much of their lives standing around.

injuries, even if relatively minor, take time to recover, since these structures are constantly in use in any upright activity. Depending on severity and other factors, recovery times of four to six weeks are not uncommon, and in cases of re-injury, much longer periods are often required. Skilled hands-on work can facilitate the recovery process, this will be discussed in greater detail in the techniques described in this chapter.

Hamstring bones, or springs?

Not only do hamstrings work hard, but they also often *feel* hard. Hamstrings are notoriously tight, and sometimes seem impervious to all attempts to lengthen them. Their resilience may be related to their function – we use them as postural muscles whenever upright, and connective tissue resilience is much more efficient than muscular contraction when continuous tension is needed. Turkeys take this a step further by developing ossifications within their leg muscles. Like us, turkeys are bipeds that spend a great deal of time standing around (Figure 9.3). To better accommodate the demands of standing, turkeys have intermuscular septa and tendons within their leg muscles that often ossify into long, thin intramuscular bonelike structures.

Although our own human hamstrings may sometimes feel as if they have ossified, their function is both to resist stretching and to spring back. Researchers such as Robert Schleip (2) and Serge Gracovetsky (3) have each described models of gait and movement based on the soft tissue's ability to store and release energy via elastic recoil. Schleip writes about how kangaroos hop much farther and faster than can be explained by the contractile force of their hamstring and leg muscles alone. Kangaroos (Figure 9.4) use a kind of "catapult effect" to load and unload their springy leg tendons (4). Rather than relying solely on muscular contraction in order to jump, kangaroos use the springiness of their leg

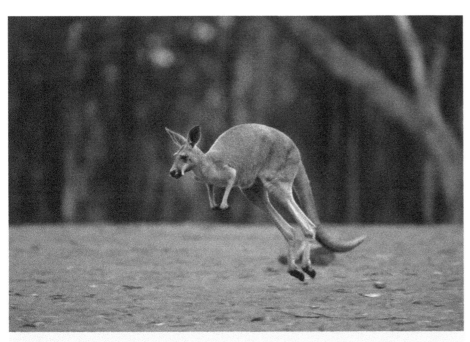

Figure 9.4

Kangaroos jump farther and faster than can be explained by muscular contraction alone – their leg tendons elastically stretch and recoil to store and release energy.

tendons to store the energy of landing, releasing it into the next hop.

These spring-like mechanisms have also been observed in antelope and humans. Ultrasound observation of human muscle during use (in this case, during oscillatory loading motions such as hopping or jumping) shows greater-than-expected tendon stretch and recoil, and less-than-expected muscle fiber shortening. Instead of shortening, muscle fibers were observed to isometrically stiffen, thereby tuning and pre-tensioning the springy tendons. One study (5) showed that 66 to 76 percent of the work involved in jumping was accomplished by stored energy within the tendinous portion of the calf's muscle-tendon complex, with only 24 to 34 percent originating from muscle contraction itself. Other fibrous connective tissues, including aponeuroses and intermuscular septa, likely contribute similar spring-like functions.

Hamstrings do not work alone; they function in concert with other myofascial and connective structures, both nearby and elsewhere in the body. The hamstrings are links in the long chains of fascial relationships that include the sacrotuberous ligament (which is aligned with the biceps femoris, sometimes sharing the same collagen fibers, and acting as a continuation of the hamstrings' force vector). In a typical cross-stride in walking or running, the gluteus maximus, the lumbodorsal fascia, and the opposite-side latissimus dorsi continue this line of connection into the contralateral arm.

The hamstrings work with other muscle groups in a variety of ways. In walking and running, the hamstrings decelerate and control the lower leg's kick-through, caused by the strong contraction of the quadriceps. One leg's hamstring muscles can all contract together, producing the powerful stride of hip extension combined with knee flexion (Figure 9.5). Conversely, the muscles can work individually, as they do when stabilizing and balancing the femur on the tibia, or when controlling tibial rotation at the bent knee, such as when changing direction while running, skiing, or skating.

When there is a lack of differentiation between the hamstrings' muscles—that is, when they are mechanically or functionally stuck together as a result of injury, overuse, habit, or unrefined body awareness – these fine-tuning functions are lost in all-or-nothing activation of the hamstrings' undifferentiated mass. This lack of differentiation can extend beyond the hamstrings, as the gluteals or adductors will sometimes fire along with hamstrings in unnecessary parasitic contractions that rob energy and reduce range. Without these functional and structural distinctions between the individual heads of the hamstrings, and between the hamstrings and its neighbors, there is dramatically reduced efficiency and a significant loss of the fine control needed for responsiveness, balance, and adaptability.

I will describe one method for increasing hamstring resilience, differentiation, and refined proprioception – the three qualities that lend spring, flow, and control to a stride.

Hamstring Technique

We will work with the client in a prone position, but some considerations are in order first. We want the client's neck to be comfortable, so using a face cradle is logical; however, most face cradles require the use of a bolster under the ankles to avoid external hip rotation or knee discomfort. This bolstered leg position does not allow full knee extension, and we want the full range of knee motion available during this technique. Rather than a built-in face cradle and a bolster under the legs, I prefer a full-torso bolster system with a table-top headrest; this allows the

client's feet to be off the table. This enables us to work the hamstrings through the full range of knee flexion and extension (Figures 9.5–9.6).

Using the flat of your forearm, begin by anchoring the outer layers of the posterior thigh (Figures 9.5 and 9.6) in a superior or proximal direction. As in the arm (see Chapter 3, the Antebrachial Fascia Technique), these surface layers include the skin, superficial fascias, and the fascia lata, the deeper fascia around and between the thigh muscles themselves. All these tissue layers tend to be thick, strong, and resilient. These tissue sheets can become adhered to one another, and to the underlying epimysial fascia around the muscles themselves.

Avoid oil or other lubricants at this point, as you will want to be able to anchor the layers in order to help them slide over one another, rather than simply sliding over the surface with your forearm. Once you have anchored the outermost of these layers, ask your client to bend his or her knee. This will allow you to move the outer layer farther in a proximal direction, effectively taking up the slack in the tissues as the knee is actively bent. No sliding on the surface has occurred yet.

Since the hamstrings are so strong and resilient, we will use the client's active movement, rather than trying to do all the work ourselves. Once the knee is fully bent (Figure 9.5), ask your client to slowly lower the leg, straightening the knee (Figure 9.6), as you allow the tissues to gradually slide out from under your forearm as they release. Even clients with hair on their legs will be comfortable if you coach them to go slowly enough. You can modulate the intensity of the release by varying your pressure and angle, and by slowing your client's motions down even further. Your client may report a mild burning or stretching; this is the sensation of the highly innervated fascial layers increasing their differentiation and elasticity. The sensation should

See video of the Hamstring Technique at http://advanced-trainings.com/v/lc06.html

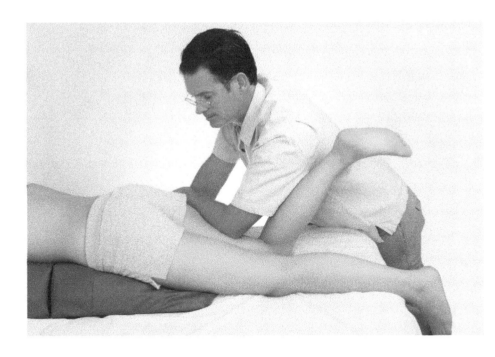

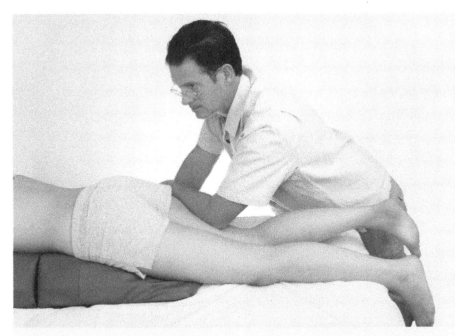

Figures 9.5/9.6

The Hamstring Technique uses the client's active lowering of the leg (knee extension) to glide and eccentrically release the tissues beneath the practitioner's static forearm. Work layer-by-layer, beginning with the superficial fascia, and continue pass by pass all the way to the intramuscular septa between the hamstrings' muscle bundles

never be so painful or intense that your client cannot relax. Repeat this release of the superficial layers in several areas of the posterior thigh – first medially, then centrally and laterally, from the ischium to the back of the knee. Your goal is a smooth, fluid sliding of the layers upon each other.

After you have worked through the outer layers, you can begin to anchor deeper structures, still working gradually and guiding your client's slow, focused movement. Remember, the release happens during the straightening of the knee, as the hamstrings' tissues and muscles are lengthened in an eccentric pattern. Feel for and differentiate between the three or four muscle bundles of the hamstrings themselves (Figure 9.7), which originate on the ischium and then split to reach around the gastrocnemius insertions at the back of the knee. In most cases, the short head of the biceps femoris crosses only the knee joint, and so it does not usually extend the hip.

Continue working on the connective tissues between and around the myofascial bundles, rather than just on the muscles' bellies. Remember that strain injuries are most common where tendon meets muscle, or where tendon meets bone. Use caution and sensitivity in the popliteal space, or in any areas where your client reports a nervy or shooting sensation (since the sciatic nerve is here as well).

In addition to hamstring injuries, other conditions will respond to direct work here. The sciatic nerve passes under the biceps femoris (Figure 9.7), where its tethering can be one cause of sciatic pain (6). Pes anserinus bursa inflammation (felt as burning and pain medial to the knee with exercise) can often be relieved by working the semitendinosus muscle, along with the gracilis and sartorius. Working the entire hamstring in the way described here can sometimes help ameliorate hamstring syndrome (a painful irritation

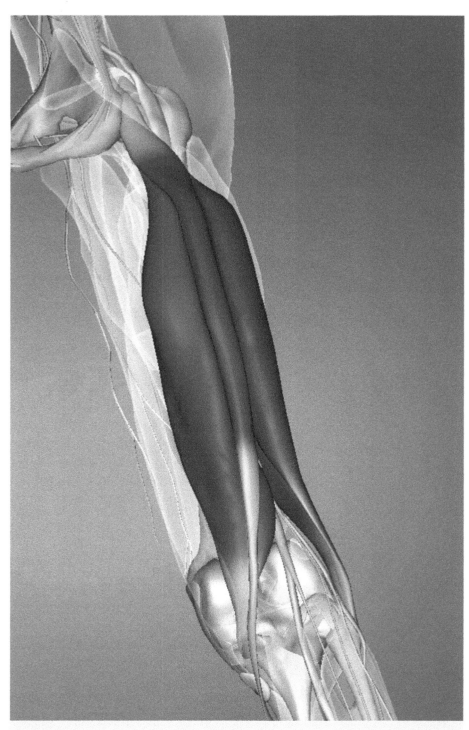

Figure 9.7
Hamstrings, medial view. Note the passage of the sciatic nerve (yellow).

of the hamstrings' attachments on the ischial tuberosity, which is often worsened by sitting).

Key points: Hamstring Technique

Indications include:
- Hamstring injury, pain, or stiffness; limited hip flexion.

Purpose
- Differentiate and increase elasticity of hamstring and posterior thigh myofascia.

Instructions
- Use forearm to anchor the fascia of the posterior thigh. Use client's slow and deliberate active knee extension to pull these tissues past your static forearm as the muscles eccentrically lengthen underneath.
- Repeat at progressively deeper layers, differentiating the heads of the hamstrings once the outer layers have been worked.

Movements
- Slow active knee extension.

Considerations for working with irritated hamstrings

As mentioned, hamstring injuries are frequently re-aggravated or kept in a state of painful irritation by overuse before they are fully healed. Ultimately, there is probably no substitute for the passage of time, and patience is sometimes the client's greatest challenge, especially for athletes who are used to pushing past the barriers. However, contrary to the conventional wisdom that says "do not do direct work on inflamed tissue," many people find that the kind of specific work described here can reduce the pain of strained tissues, and this can accelerate the recovery process, even when applied directly to inflamed and painful areas. There is good research-based evidence showing that hands-on manipulation can reduce exercise-induced inflammation. One study found significant reductions in chemical markers of inflammation in leg tissues after massage (7). Another study found fewer adhesions between the layers of connective tissue when manual manipulation was performed on mechanically irritated tissues (8). If you and your client do decide to try these techniques directly on painful areas, the suggested protocol would be to do a small amount of this work, and wait 2–3 days to see how the hamstrings respond. If there was no change, or an overall reduction in pain, irritation, or stiffness after 2–3 days (even if the initial reaction was the opposite), then you can safely try a bit more direct work at the next session. If, on the other hand, there was increased irritation or stiffness with no resulting improvement, work elsewhere or in different ways, rather than continue using the same techniques.

There are several theories about the actual mechanism by which hands-on work helps injured tissues. Examples of these are improved tissue hydration, stimulation of collagen renewal, better organization of newly forming collagen, trigger-point prevention, increased proprioceptive accuracy, and interruption of self-perpetuating pain cycles. Although not all of these models have been tested via formal research yet, any of them can provide practitioners with a useful mental map for conceptualizing what they may be achieving with their work. No matter which model makes the most sense to you (and fits best with your style, experience, viewpoint, and population served), chances are you will find plenty of opportunity to use hamstring techniques in your practice.

References

[1] Heiderscheit, B. et al. (2010) Hamstring strain injuries: recommendations for diagnosis, rehabilitation and injury prevention. *Journal of Orthopaedic & Sports Physical Therapy.* 40(2). p. 67–81.

[2] Müller, D. and Schleip, R. (2012). Fascial fitness: Suggestions for a fascia-oriented training approach in sports and movement therapies. in *Fascia, The Tensional Network of the Human Body.* 7(254). p. 465

[3] Gracovetsky, S. (2003) *The Spinal Engine.* UK: Springer.

[4] Kram, R. and Dawson, T.J. (1998) Energetics and Biomechanics of Locomotion by Red Kangaroos (Macropus rufus). *Comparative Biochemistry & Physiology.* 120(1). p. 41–49 [accessed December 2013, http:// stripe.colorado.edu/~kram/kangaroo.pdf]

[5] American Society of Biomechanics, T. Fukunaga et al. (2001) Muscle Fiber Behavior During Drop Jump in Humans. www.asbweb.org/conferences/2001/pdf/168.pdf. [Accessed November 2013]

[6] Saikku, K. et al. (2010): Entrapment of the Proximal Sciatic Nerve by the Hamstring Tendons. *Acta Orthopaedica Belgica.* 76. p. 321–324.

[7] Crane, J.D. et al. (2012) Massage Therapy Attenuates Inflammatory Signaling After Exercise-Induced Muscle Damage. *Science Translational Medicine.* 4(119).

[8] Bove, G.M. and Chapelle, S.L. (2012) Visceral Mobilization can Lyse and Prevent Peritoneal Adhesions in a Rat Model," *Journal of Bodywork & Movement Therapies.* 16(1). p. 76–82.

Figure credits

Figures 9.1 and 9.7 courtesy Primal Pictures, used by permission.
Figure 9.2 modified from an image by Hellerhoff, used under CCA-SA 3.0.
Figures 9.3 and 9.4 courtesy Thinkstock.
Figures 9.5 and 9.6 courtesy Advanced-Trainings.com, used by permission.

Study Guide

Hamstring Injuries

1 The text states that the most frequently injured hamstring muscle is the:

a semitendinosus
b semimembranosus
c quadratus femoris
d biceps femoris

2 The text states that the two most common sites for hamstring injury are the musculotendinous junctions, and the:

a distal attachment of the semitendinosus
b distal attachment of the semimembranosus
c ischial tuberosity
d distal attachment of the quadratus femoris

3 What structure does the text say is aligned with the biceps femoris, and acts as a continuation of that hamstring's force vector?

a IT band
b lateral gastrocnemius
c gluteus maximus
d sacrotuberous ligament

4 When the hamstrings lose structural or functional differentiation, which of the following does the text state will sometimes fire in unison with them?

a gluteals
b quads
c psoas
d hip abductors

5 The Hamstring Technique utilizes which active client movement:

a knee flexion
b knee extension
c hip extension
d ankle plantarflexion

For Answer Keys, visit www.Advanced-Trainings.com/v1key/

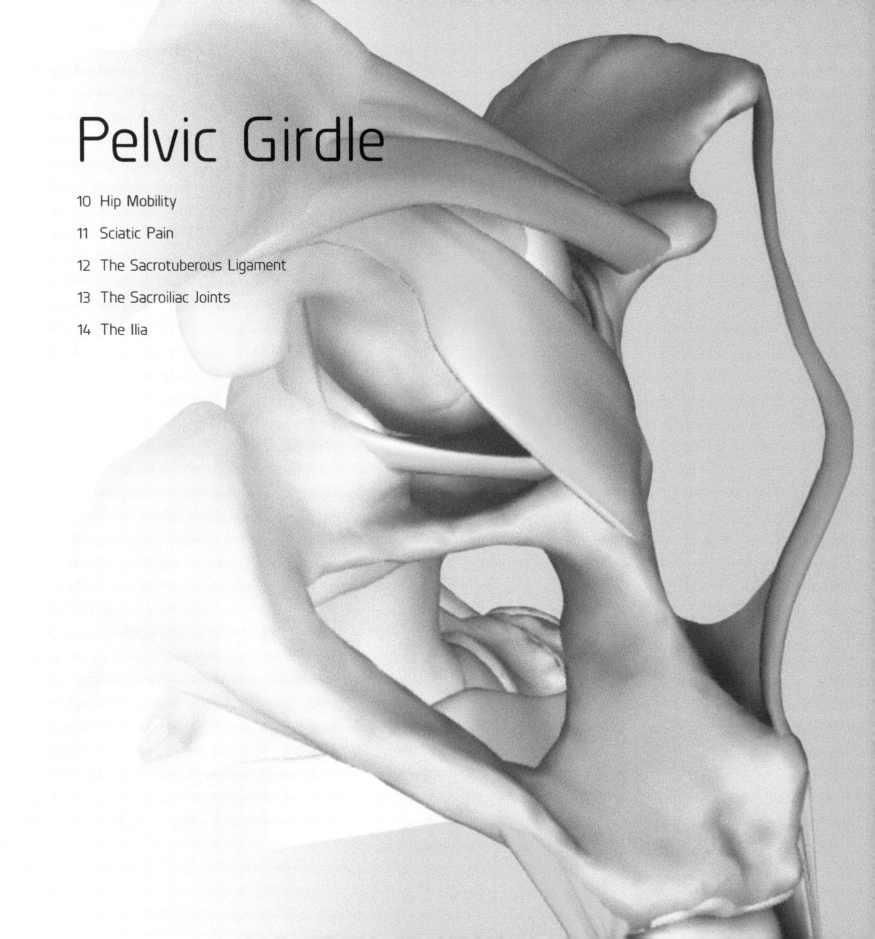

Pelvic Girdle

Hip Mobility

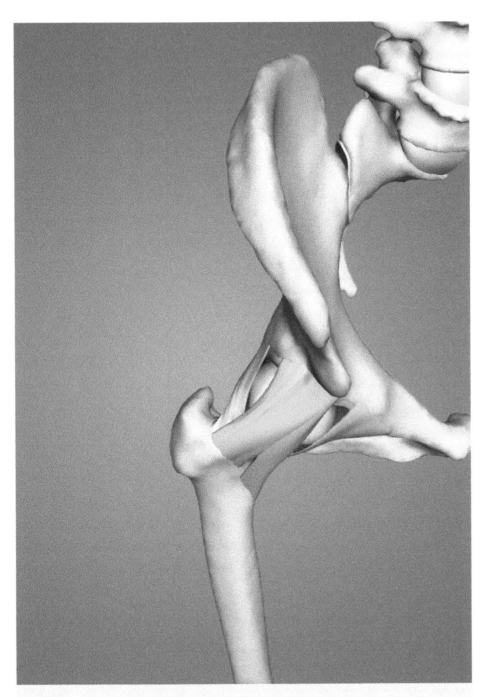

Figure 10.1
The iliofemoral, pubofemoral, and ischiofemoral ligaments limit hip motion.

When I was a student at the Rolf Institute in the 1980s, I heard a story about its founder, Dr. Ida Rolf, which underlined the importance of pelvic mobility in her work. According to the story, Dr. Rolf would regularly quiz her trainees about the aims of each of her ten "hours" or sessions.

She reportedly asked her classes questions such as, "What is the goal of the fifth hour?" As a demanding teacher, very few answers would satisfy her; but even though each session was different, she reportedly accepted the answer "free the pelvis" as a correct one, no matter which session she would ask about.

While this story probably has an element of folklore to it (since her death in 1979, many "Ida stories" have assumed the status of legend in the structural integration community), it illustrates the key role that pelvic adaptability at the hip joints played in her vision of an integrated body. Dr. Rolf referred to the hips and pelvis as "the joint that determines symmetry." She was not alone in emphasizing the key role of the hips; balanced hip joint mobility is important in fields as diverse as athletics, dance, geriatrics, and back pain management.

I became even more curious about the relationship of the low back to hip-joint mobility when I traveled to Japan to teach and practice manual therapy, a few years after graduating from the Rolf Institute. I noticed challenges in my own hip mobility as I adjusted to the Japanese practice of sitting on floor cushions more often than on chairs. I noticed considerably more hip mobility (especially external rotation) in my Japanese clientele than I had seen in my American and European clients.

My Japanese clients also seemed to have generally flatter spinal curves. Was this also related to their hip mobility? In utero, humans develop with flexed hips and no secondary lumbar curve

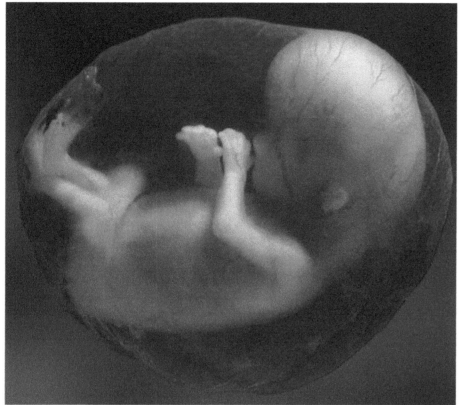

Watch Til Luchau demonstrate the Push Broom techniques: http://advanced-trainings.com/v/pa04.html

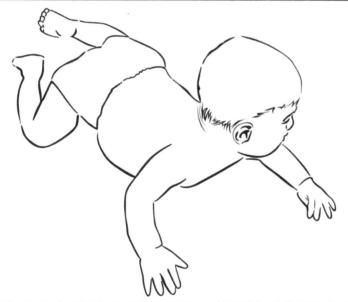

Figures 10.2/10.3

Infants have more hip flexion as a result of their position in utero.

(Figure 10.2). It is only once they begin to crawl (Figure 10.3) and extend their hips that they develop a lumbar curve. Conventional wisdom maintains that freer hips mean happier backs, and research both in Japan (1) and in the USA (2) generally supports this.

In this chapter, I will describe three techniques that are used to assess and balance hip joint mobility, which can be useful when working not only with hip mobility issues directly, but as a way to ameliorate low back pain and other issues.

Techniques

Push Broom "A" Technique

The "Push Broom" series is an effective way to increase hip joint mobility without undue effort or strain by the practitioner. Using gravity, we will take the hip through three positional techniques that will release all of the structures in the hip joint: from the deep iliofemoral ligaments (Figure 10.1), to the iliopsoas, hamstrings, hip abductors and adductors, rotators, sartorius, quadriceps, and their enveloping fascias.

The term "push broom" refers to the starting grip: hold your prone client's leg at the ankle and knee as if holding the handle of a push broom (Figure 10.4). Swing the knee outwards as you walk the leg up into full hip flexion, bringing the knee as far towards the head as comfortably possible. Rolling the pelvis away from you as you bring the knee up will make it easier to flex the hip past the 90-degree point. With almost all clients, it will be more comfortable if you take the leg past this 90-degree position so that the femur is close to the side of the body, rather than perpendicular to it.

Simply being put into this "baby crawling" or "bullfrog" position often gives a therapeutic stretch to the hip joints; however, while we are here, we can increase hip mobility by

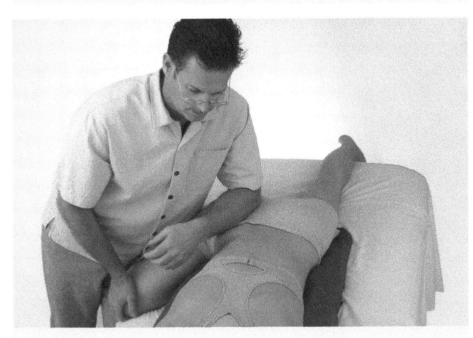

Figure 10.4
The "A" variation of the Push Broom Technique.

Figure 10.5
Once the hip is flexed with the lower leg on the table, use your forearms to release the medial attachments of the gluteal muscles.

releasing the gluteals. While stabilizing your client's leg with your own, use the flat of your forearm to gently lean into the medial attachments of the gluteus maximus just below the iliac crest (Figures 10.5 and 10.6). Tendinous attachments have concentrations of Golgi tendon organs. These respond to sustained pressure, so you will get the best results by waiting with slow, nearly static pressure here, rather than sliding or moving your touch. Use moderate pressure, with a slight vector of pressure towards yourself, in order to ease or nudge the gluteus away from its bony attachments on the ilium.

Gently sustain this pressure until you feel the tissue respond with a subtle softening or easing; then, release your pressure and move to the next segment of gluteal attachments.

Key points: Push Broom Techniques

Indications include:
- Limited hip mobility.
- Balance or gait issues.
- Back, sacroiliac, or sciatic pain.

Purpose
- Restore mobility and refine proprioception at the iliofemoral (hip) joint.

Instructions
- Without causing any pain, gently bring leg into flexed, abducted and rotated positions as described in the text. Use static pressure on muscle attachments.
- Wait in each position for a tissue response to the stretch.
- Repeat with other hip.

For almost all clients, the position is more comfortable when taken past 90 degrees of flexion.

Cautions
- Certain movements may be contraindicated for recent hip replacement patients.

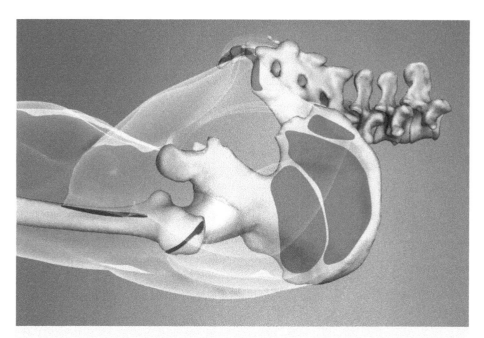

Figure 10.6
The medial attachments of the gluteus muscles.

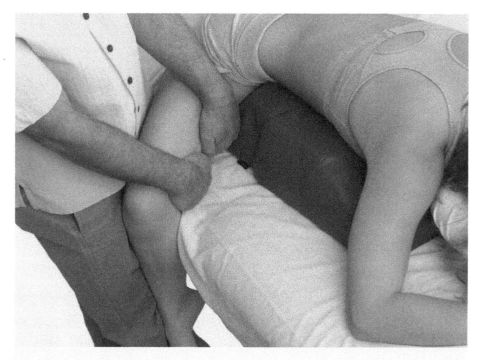

Figure 10.7
The "B" (external rotation) variation of the Push Broom Technique.

Push Broom "B" (External Rotation)

While still in the leg-up position of the Push Broom "A" technique, drop your client's lower leg off the table (Figure 10.7). Roll the femur into external rotation by lifting the adductors towards you with both hands. This also allows you to prevent any pressure that the edge of the table might otherwise put behind your client's knee. At the same time, use your leg under the table to augment the femoral rotation by gently pressing your client's foot towards the head of the table. Your client should feel no strain on the knee or anywhere else – only a stretch and release around the hip joint (Figure 10.8). Omit the pressure on your client's foot if it produces any discomfort.

Stay comfortable and upright in your own body. Invite your client to breathe easily and relax into the stretch. Sustain this positional technique until you feel a response – softening, easing, or relaxing. Usually this takes at least three to five breaths.

Push Broom "C" (Internal Rotation)

Specific kinds of hip mobility have been correlated with low back health. Internal hip rotation, hip flexion, and hip extension in both sexes, and hamstring flexibility in men, all have a negative correlation with back pain (that is, people with those types of mobility generally have less back pain) (3). The "C" variation of the Push Broom Technique combines several of these important motions: internal femoral rotation, hip flexion, and hamstring stretch.

From the external rotation "B" variation, go right into internal rotation with Push Broom "C". Instead of dropping the lower leg below the level of the table as in "B", rotate the femur so that the lower leg is high. By using the grip and position shown in Figure 10.9, gently take the femur to its soft end-range of internal rotation; hold, and wait for tissue response. Remember to keep the

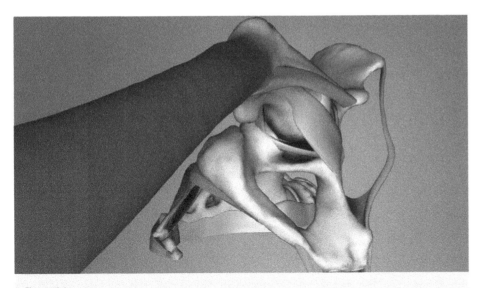

Figure 10.8
Viewing the hip joint from below helps visualize how external rotation can open the anterior hip joint.

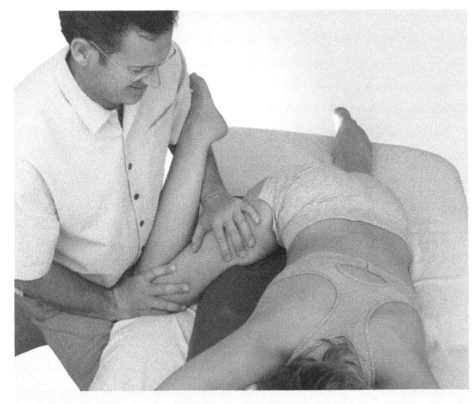

Figure 10.9
The "C" variation of the Push Broom Technique (internal rotation).

hip flexed at least 90 degrees (that is, keep the femur perpendicular to the body, or even a little past this position toward the head). As in the "B" variation, be mindful to avoid strain or discomfort on the knee.

Once you have completed these three Push Broom variations on one leg, return the leg to its anatomical position. Clients will often comment that this leg feels significantly longer and freer than the one you have not yet worked on. Repeat these techniques with the other side to balance the left and right sides.

Other considerations

Although we have described these three variations above as hip joint techniques, they also affect the ligamentous adaptability of the pelvic girdle itself, mobilizing the sacroiliac joints by addressing sacrotuberous, sacrospinous, and sacroiliac ligament restrictions, and balancing the torsion and flaring movements of the ilia on the sacrum. This makes them useful in addressing appendicular sciatic pain (Chapter 11), sacrotuberous pain (Chapter 12), sacroiliac pain (Chapter 13), and other conditions of the pelvis.

If your client or patient is unclothed or minimally clothed, you can drape these techniques by simply grasping the leg through the top sheet in variation "A", and move the sheet together with the leg. Alternatively, especially for the "B" and "C" variations, the leg can be out of the drape, with the sheet gathered around the thigh so as to give a sense of security and privacy to the client.

When applying the techniques described here, it is important that they do not cause pain. In addition to soft-tissue restrictions to mobility, there can be bony restrictions as well, such as the shape or orientation of the acetabula or femoral heads. These can cause pain or irritation when pushed to their physiologic limit. Femoral acetabular impingement (FAI) syndrome is a painful restriction of hip movement caused by

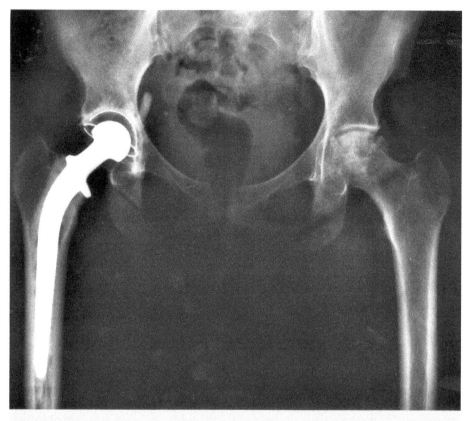

Figure 10.10

X-ray of a total hip replacement (total hip arthroplasty)

abnormal contact between the femur and the rim of the acetabulum, probably due to both genetic and usage factors. Although often addressed surgically, techniques that increase mobility are also effective in managing FAI pain –though pushing a stretch too aggressively can aggravate this condition, so use caution at the end ranges of motion, especially if there is discomfort deep in the hip joint itself.

What about hip replacements?

Although the prevention of difficulties is more difficult to measure or study than the difficulties themselves, it is reasonable to assume that maintaining balanced hip mobility can help prevent or ameliorate the joint pain, degeneration, or arthritic conditions that if otherwise unaddressed, can lead to hip replacement or resurfacing.

If your client has already had hip replacement surgery (Figure 10.10), special considerations may apply when using these techniques. Hip replacement surgery involves cutting through tissues and dislocating the joint being replaced, either posteriorly or anteriorly, depending on the type of surgery. This can leave the hip with less support in the direction of the surgical dislocation, at least during recovery.[1]

Different types of hip surgeries have different movement restrictions associated with their recovery period. Surgeons also differ widely in their recommended movement restrictions after surgery. In 2010, during an informal survey of hip surgeons' recommendations to yoga teachers, it was found that a third of responding surgeons did not require any movement restrictions whatsoever after an anterior hip replacement (4). However, the most conservative recommendations say that for six months to one year after surgery, hip replacement patients should avoid:

---

1 To learn more about the procedures involved in a posterior replacement, I recommend checking out edhead.org's interactive hip surgery simulator at www.edheads.org/activities/hip/. The squeamish need not be concerned – the animated procedures keep it neat and tidy, unlike real posterior hip surgeries, which can appear downright gory and brutal to the uninitiated. Accessed 5/2014.

- Adduction, internal rotation, and hip flexion past 90 degrees for posterior hip replacements
- Abduction, external rotation, and hip extension for anterior replacements.

Given these variables, the best practice for manual therapists is to inquire about any movements that the client's surgeon or rehabilitation therapist recommended avoiding during the recovery period.

Many hip replacement patients continue to experience soft tissue-based movement restrictions long after their surgeries have fully healed. For these older, healed hip replacements (approximately one year or more after surgery), these techniques can be a great help with longer-term recovery and maintenance of mobility. However, given that we are not trying to stretch or alter the artificial materials of the prosthesis itself, go easy on the end-range of any stretching applied to the replaced hip. Think about keeping the tissues around the joint long, easy, and mobile, rather than trying to deeply stretch the artificial joint itself.

Finally, do not hesitate to adapt these techniques for senior or physically challenged clients. By being sensitive and staying in communication about their comfort, you will often be surprised as to how comfortable and effective these releases are, even for those with limited active mobility.

With practice, these techniques will become indispensable parts of your technique toolbox, enabling you to assess and release many hip restrictions within the context of your regular work. Your clients of all ages and activity levels will appreciate this: whether we have lower back pain or not (and 80 percent of people experience back pain at some point in their lives), most of us will benefit from increased hip adaptability, as it makes our sitting, walking, and moving easier, more efficient, and more comfortable.

References

[1] Horikawa, K. et al. (2006) Prevalence of osteoarthritis, osteoporotic vertebral fractures, and spondylolisthesis among the elderly in a Japanese village. *Journal of Orthopaedic Surgery.* 14(1). p. 9–12.

[2] Harris-Hayes, M. et al. (2009) Relationship between the hip and low back pain in athletes who participate in rotation-related sports. *Journal of Sport Rehabilitation.* Feb; 18(1) p. 60–75.

[3] Mellin, G. (1988) Correlations of hip mobility with degree of back pain and lumbar spinal mobility in chronic low-back pain patients. *Spine.* 13(6) p. 668–670.

[4] Jones, N.M. (2010) *Yoga after a Hip Replacement.* http://www.xpandinglight.org/free/yoga-teacher/articles/yoga-therapy/yoga-after-a-hip-replacement.asp. [Accessed 5/2014]

Picture credits

Figures 10.1, 10.6 and 10.8 courtesy Primal Pictures, used by permission.
Figure 10.2 is a public domain image.
Figures 10.3, 10.4, 10.5, 10.7 and 10.9 courtesy Advanced-Trainings.com, used by permission.
Figures 10.10 is a public domain image from the National Institutes of Health.

Study Guide

Hip Mobility

1 The text cites research that indicates that freer hips correlate with:

a less knee pain
b less back pain
c less shoulder pain
d less jaw pain

2 Which types of hip mobility have been correlated with low back health in both men and women?

a external hip rotation, hip flexion and extension
b internal hip rotation, hip flexion and extension
c internal hip rotation, hip flexion and hip abduction
d external hip rotation, hip flexion and hip adduction

3 In the Push Broom "A" Technique, the practitioner applies static pressure to the attachments of the gluteus maximus:

a just above the iliac crest
b just below the iliac crest
c at the ischial tuberosity
d the gluteus maximus attachment to the ITT

4 The author states that the Golgi tendon organs located in the tendinous attachments respond best to:

a sliding pressure
b pulsing pressure
c light pressure
d sustained pressure

5 The text suggests holding the position of the Push Broom "B" Technique:

a 3–5 minutes
b 3–5 breaths
c 3–5 seconds
d 3–5 times

For Answer Keys, visit www.Advanced-Trainings.com/v1key/

Sciatic Pain

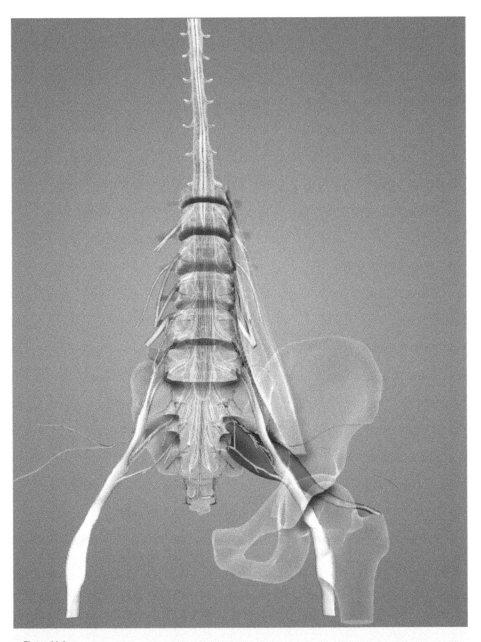

Figure 11.1

The origins of the sciatic nerve – the largest and longest nerve in the body. Pain results when its nerve roots are compressed where they exit the lumbar spine (axial sciatica) or when it is entrapped distally by other structures (appendicular sciatica). The dura (aqua color), psoas (green), and piriformis (red) are some of the structures that can contribute to sciatic pain.

Sciatica is a real pain in the rear – not just for the individuals who experience it, but collectively, for society as a whole. Although estimates vary, studies indicate that up to 43 percent of people experience sciatic pain at some point in their lives (1). A 2008 meta-analysis of sciatic studies concluded that sciatic pain is more persistent, more severe, and consumes even more health resources than low back pain does (2).

Sciatica can also be a pain for manual therapy practitioners. Sometimes, sciatic pain responds quickly; at other times, it seems intractable, and it can even worsen in response to hands-on work. As a practitioner, how do you determine which approaches are most likely to be helpful? In this chapter, we will take a look at straightforward and relatively reliable assessments for differentiating between the two types of sciatic pain; we will discuss important considerations for working with the first (axial) type; and we will describe the techniques and approaches used for relieving the second (appendicular) type.

Much of sciatica's ubiquity and variability comes from the broadness of the term. Originally derived from "ischialgia," meaning pelvic or ischium pain, sciatica has come to mean any pain involving the lower back or buttocks that radiates down the posterior leg. Sciatica is a symptom, not a diagnosis; there are many possible causes of sciatic pain, and knowing how to distinguish between its different types will allow you to be far more effective in your work (and it will help you to know when to refer to a specialist).

One thing is common to all sciatic pain: it is nerve pain, and so it can be radiating, shooting, sharp, tingling, or numb. Sciatic pain involves an irritating mechanical force on a nerve, usually somewhere along the neurons (nerve cells) that

	Axial Sciatica	Appendicular Sciatica
Also known as...	Type I, "TRUE SCIATICA"	Type II, "PSEUDOSCIATICA", Piriformis Syndrome, etc.
Entrapment site	Nerve roots	Distal to nerve roots
Entrapment mechanism	Bone-to-bone or disc-to-bone compression	Myofascial compression or neurofascial tethering
Low back pain	Usually present	Usually absent
Posterior thigh and/or buttock pain	Usually present	Usually present
Pain distal to knee	Usually absent	Sometimes present

Table 11.1 Types of sciatic pain. In addition to the mechanisms of entrapment listed above, infection, tumors, and direct trauma (either at the nerve roots or distally) can also cause nerve entrapment and sciatic symptoms.

make up the sciatic nerve (usually because irritation of the other nerves can sometimes radiate to the sciatic nerve distribution area as well).

Assessing sciatic pain

Sciatic pain can be described as one of two types, as outlined in Table 11.1:

I. Axial sciatica arises from compression on the nerve roots at the intervertebral foramina of nerves L1–S3[1] (3).

II. Appendicular sciatica is pain from nerve entrapment distal to the nerve roots.

The first type, axial sciatica, involves narrowing of the foramina (the openings between the vertebra where the peripheral nerves exit the spinal canal (Figures 11.1, 11.2 and 11.9). This narrowing can result from:

- Postural or positional issues – for example, the postural strain of later-term pregnancy, sacral instability, or spondylolisthesis (the instability and anterior shift of a vertebra on the one below it, narrowing their intervertebral foramen)
- Articular disc degeneration, herniation, or bulging into the foraminal space
- Stenosis (bony deposits in the foramen or spinal canal).

These mechanisms involve compression of the nerve roots between the adjacent vertebrae (bone-to-bone compression) or between a disc and vertebra (disc-to-bone). There are also reports of small accessory muscles being found within the foramen parallel to the nerves (4), as well as dural tube adhesions at the nerve roots – either of which could conceivably cause axial sciatic pain. Infections, tumors, cancer, or trauma at the nerve roots (or elsewhere along the nerve) can also cause sciatic pain, and they are the reasons why referral to a specialist is prudent when sciatic pain is persistent, unresponsive, or severe.

1 The sciatic nerve itself has components from nerves L4-S3; however, impingements of L1-L3 have been observed to cause sciatic-type symptoms as well.

Axial sciatica will show one or more of these signs:

- Pain in the low back along with buttock or thigh pain, usually without pain below the knee (unless there are also appendicular contributors)[2]

- "Sciatic scoliosis": a reluctance to put weight on the affected side, resulting in leaning away from the affected side in order to minimize pain.

- A positive (i.e., painful) result when performing the Straight Leg Test.

Straight Leg Test

The Straight Leg Test (SLT) or the Lasègue Test is a common and reasonably reliable assessment for identifying lumbar nerve root compression. With your client seated at the front edge of a chair, ask him or her to raise a straightened leg at the hip (that is, with his or her knee extended straight). The straight leg test is positive (meaning that it indicates likely nerve root compression) if sciatic pain is reproduced with the motions listed in the caption of Figure 11.3. Pain in the opposite (supporting) leg can be due to more severe disc herniation, and is clear cause for referral.

Why do ankle dorsiflexion, slumping, or neck flexion increase sciatic pain in the SLT when a nerve root is compressed? All three of these movements stretch the nerve tissues further, putting a little more tension on any entrapment. Slumping and neck flexion also pull upwards (caudally) on the dural tube within the spinal canal. The dural tube's projections surround the nerve roots and line each foramen (Figure 11.2), so restrictions here can be a cause of axial sciatic pain. If this is the case, the slump test itself can be a helpful self-treatment, gently stretching the dural adhesions. Clients should be instructed not to over-do the stretching, or do

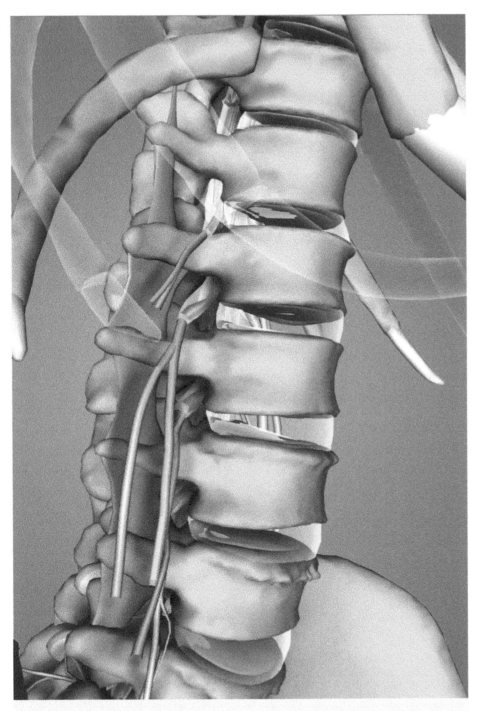

Figure 11.2

Protruding or degenerated intervertebral discs (green) or the dura (aqua color) can impinge the nerve roots where they exit the spinal canal, resulting in axial sciatic pain.

2 Although some systems teach that pain below the knee is an indication of nerve root impingement (i.e., axial sciatica), "The only pain that has ever been produced experimentally by stimulating nerve roots is shooting pain in a band-like distribution. There is no physiological evidence that constant, deep aching pain in the lower leg [below the knee] arises from nerve root irritation." (5) In my own experience, pain below the knee has usually accompanied other signs (such as a positive piriformis test, or a painfully unstable sacrum) that suggest appendicular causes, even when confirmed axial issues were present.

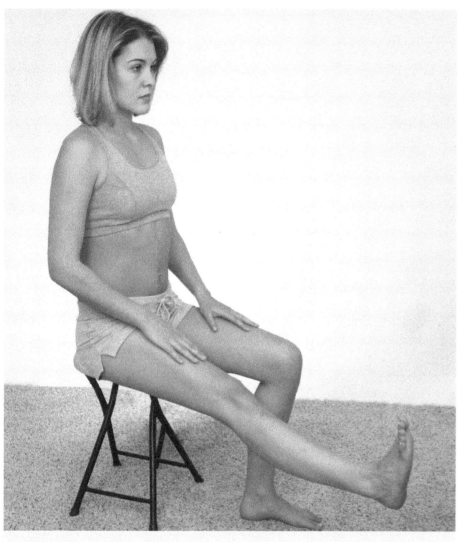

Figure 11.3

The Straight Leg Test (SLT) indicates probable nerve root compression if: 1) sciatic pain is reproduced between 30° and 70° of hip flexion (70° is pictured); 2) pain worsens with ankle dorsiflexion, slumping, or neck flexion (dropping the head forward); or 3) pain is relieved by knee flexion of the raised leg.

too many repetitions, so as to avoid aggravating the already inflamed nerve roots.

The SLT can also be performed passively, or with your client supine instead of sitting. Including these variations may increase the accuracy of your findings. Supine testing does not allow for the slump test, but it does make it easier to add the bowstring variation of the SLT (described later in this chapter), which can help determine if there is appendicular involvement in addition to axial sciatic nerve entrapment.

When performed and interpreted correctly, the SLT has a high statistical sensitivity (91 percent of correct positive results), but a lower statistical specificity (26 percent of correct negative results) (6). In other words, the SLT is quite reliable at indicating compression of the sciatic nerve roots (about nine out of ten positive results will accurately indicate nerve root involvement). However, the SLT is less reliable at determining when there is not nerve root compression (in other words, among those who have nerve root compression – as verified by other clinical means – three out of four will test negative with the SLT). In other words, the SLT is fairly good at ruling in nerve root compression, but it is fairly bad at ruling it out.

Of course, you should keep in mind that unless your training and licensing specifically permit you to diagnose conditions like disc issues, it is inappropriate to offer your client a diagnosis, or even suggest an interpretation of the SLT, for a variety of good reasons. Even if you are a physician or other licensed professional whose scope of practice does include diagnosis, telling someone with a positive SLT that they have a nine in ten chance of having a nerve root entrapment is a loaded and potentially complex conversation, with the potential for inadvertent harm as well as good. For most manual therapists, a positive SLT is reason to refer the client to a specialist for further evaluation, or to confirm that your client is already under a specialist's care. Even in these cases, knowing and using the SLT will allow you to strategize your own work appropriately.

Working with axial sciatica

Since they involve different entrapment sites and mechanisms, axial and appendicular sciatica are approached in different ways. Because many of the causes of axial sciatic pain involve instability, bone-to-bone, or whole-body patterns, direct myofascial work with axial sciatica can be quite tricky. Although there are very effective manual therapy approaches which address the lumbar causes of axial sciatic pain, they often involve skilled discernment and judicious application by an experienced practitioner. While deep lumbar work can sometimes be quite helpful for someone with axial sciatic symptoms; however, if it is performed unskillfully, deep or overly-focused work (including trigger point work, active release, deep massage, structural work, or direct myofascial release) can in some cases worsen the symptoms of lumber disc issues by inadvertently releasing the adaptations and compensations that are providing stability to an unstable spine.

For this reason, many of the actual techniques for working with axial sciatica are probably beyond the scope of a written instructional text like this one, and are best learned in an in-person training environment, followed by engaging in cautious practice while having access to experienced supervision and advice.

However, even without specialized in-person training, there is a tremendous amount of benefit that manual therapy can provide. These pointers will help increase your effectiveness while minimizing risk to your clients who show signs of axial sciatica:

1. The safest, most universally helpful intentions for manual therapists when dealing with axial sciatica are to gently ease the effects of unnecessary splinting and guarding, and to relieve the overall tension and stress of dealing with pain. Relaxing and calming approaches, such as massage therapy, as well as work around the lateral hips, shoulders, and neck, are especially helpful.

2. Work slowly. If you do deep work, proceed very gradually, noting your client's response between sessions. If there is a persistent increase in pain after your session, work less deeply next session, and/or in different places. Techniques that feel good on the table may worsen the symptoms when upright so, if possible, ask your client to sit or stand partway through your session to check in about pain level, and adjust or redirect your work accordingly.

3. Employ your client's own gentle active movements, rather than passive moving, stretching, or positioning. Use your client's comfort as a guide. Painful work is not helpful with inflammatory conditions such as sciatica, so your clients should be instructed not to push through their pain. Find a level of depth and pressure that allows your client to relax into the work.

4. Especially in cases of sciatica and other nerve issues, the point of greatest pain is often the place that is least in need of direct, deep pressure. Because tissues are already inflamed or unstable where they are most painful, direct work may worsen the symptoms later. Instead, ease the body around the most painful areas.

5. Avoid any techniques that apply longitudinal compression or shearing forces (listhesis) to the spine, such as downward pressure in a prone position, and some seated techniques or passive stretches. Also, use caution with positions or techniques that twist the spine, which can narrow the foremen around an already crowded nerve root (twists can

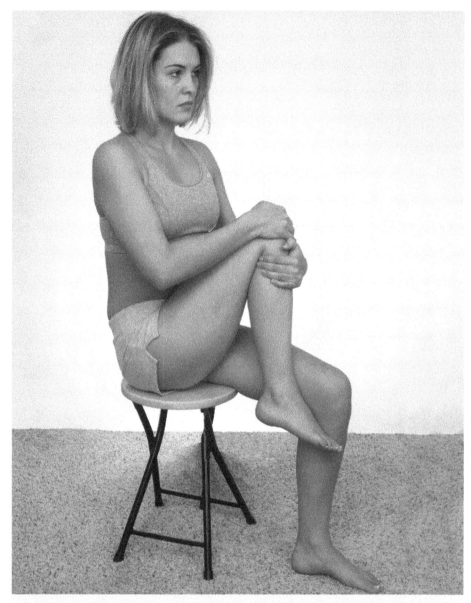

Figure 11.4

The Piriformis Test. An increase in sciatic symptoms when the flexed leg is brought across the body (adduction) indicates probable piriformis or rotator involvement. This can also be performed passively or with the client supine.

sometimes also relieve compression, but use them cautiously).

6. It is a good idea for clients with acute axial sciatic signs to be under the care of a spine specialist such as an orthopedist, chiropractor, physical therapist, or other rehabilitation specialist. If you suspect undiagnosed lumbar disc issues (for example, if your client feels a worsening of sciatic symptoms with the Straight Leg Test), be sure to refer your client to a qualified medical specialist for evaluation and possible rehabilitative work. Do not hesitate to get supervision or advice from a mentor as well.

Even with this long list of cautions, do not be discouraged. Remember that your work can dramatically help someone with axial sciatic pain. Relaxing and calming are always helpful, and easing the overall patterns of guarding and stress from chronic pain can be a godsend for someone with unrelenting sciatic pain.

Assessing appendicular sciatica

Whether or not the SLT indicates possible nerve root compression, you will want to check for distal contributions to sciatic pain to further narrow down your choice of possible techniques. Often, axial sciatica is accompanied by appendicular sciatica as well. In contrast to the bone-to-bone or disc-to-bone compression of axial sciatica, appendicular sciatica entrapment is typically related to the soft tissues, which often respond very readily to direct manual therapy. We will describe three ways of assessing appendicular sciatica: the Bowstring Variation of the SLT, the Piriformis Test, and the Sciatic Nerve Glide Test.

The Bowstring Test

The Bowstring Test is a variation of the SLT. Once you have performed the SLT and found positive (painful) results, support your seated client's

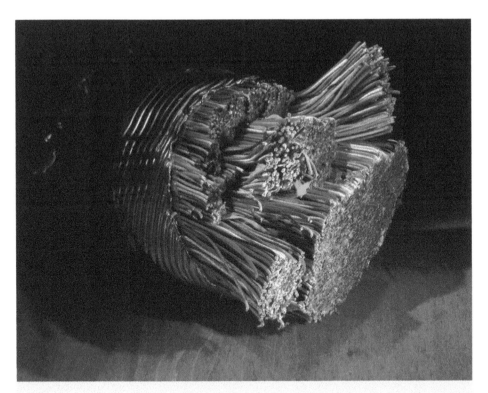

Figure 11.5

Although living nerves are much more complex than wires, a nerve's connective tissue layers are analogous to the layered wrappings around an electrical cable.

The Piriformis Test

Nerve entrapment by the piriformis muscle is the most common cause of appendicular sciatica, probably accounting for about 70 percent of all non-lumbar sciatic pain[3] so this test will help identify the most probable cause of appendicular sciatic pain (7).

To perform this test, ask your seated or supine client to pull the knee of the affected leg to his or her chest (Figure 11.4). Once the hip is flexed in this way, if actively bringing the knee across the midline of the body (adduction with flexion) increases sciatic pain, this indicates probable piriformis or hamstring entrapment of the sciatic nerve.

Assessing Sciatic Nerve Glide

Nerves are not wires. Although both nerves and wires transmit electrical impulses, nerves are much more than electrical cables (Figure 11.5). Nerves, because they are living, perceptive, and sentient structures, are sensitive to being crowded, confined, strangled, or overstretched. When the sciatic nerve is entrapped or irritated, pain in the low back, buttock, and lower limb is the result.

As described above, sciatic pain arises from either axial origins (typically at the spinal nerve roots) or from appendicular causes (distal entrapments in the buttocks, hip, or leg). Before we move on to assessing and addressing more appendicular impingements, let us take a look at nerve entrapment.

Understanding nerve entrapment

In order to understand sciatic nerve entrapment, it is helpful to review some important features about nerves in general, and the sciatic nerve in particular. The neurons that make up the sciatic nerve are the longest in the body – originating in the spinal cord and extending to the hip, leg,

hip at the angle of maximum sciatic symptoms. Slightly flexing the knee in this position usually relieves sciatic symptoms, since it slackens the tension on the sciatic nerve and its roots. To check for peripheral sciatic nerve involvement (appendicular sciatica), apply gentle but firm pressure with your thumbs or fingers into the popliteal space, with a slight distal traction on the tissue around the nerve (similar to the Sciatic Nerve Traction technique shown in Figures 11.19 and 11.20). Since the sciatic nerve is here at the back of the knee, pain with pressure or traction indicates peripheral sciatic nerve involvement due to localized stretch of the nerve and nerve sheath.

3 Researchers at Cedars-Sinai Medical Center; the University of California, Los Angeles; and the Institute for Nerve Medicine in Los Angeles examined 2239 sciatic patients (using magnetic resonance neurography) who hadn't improved with lumbar disc treatment. Results of the study confirmed that 69 percent had piriformis syndrome, while the remaining 31 percent had a combination of other nerve, SI joint or muscle conditions.

3. give the nerve its structure, tensile resilience, and elasticity.

Impingement (compression or tension) on the nerve impairs all three of these functions, causing internal inflammation of the nerve, reducing its blood flow, and diminishing its ability to glide and stretch.

The third quality, elastic glide, is particularly relevant to our work. In an average sized adult, the long neurons within the sciatic nerve stretch an additional 3.5 to 5 inches with normal hip, knee, and ankle motions (8). This causes a significant amount of gliding movement between the epineurium and the surrounding intermuscular septa, muscle sheathes, and supporting fascias. A nerve gliding within these surrounding connective tissues can be compared to a tendon's movement within its surrounding bursa. As with other fascia and connective tissues, the epineurium sheath around a nerve may itself become adhered or tethered to surrounding structures (losing differentiation); it may also become hardened and thickened from strain or injury (losing elasticity). Since this protective sheath contains blood vessels that supply the nerve (Figure 11.6), adhesions or hardening of the epineurium can choke the nerve's circulation, worsening the internal inflammation.

Impingements on the nerve sheath may also cause pain directly; the sheath itself is highly enervated by smaller sensory nerve filaments (the nervi nervorum) that are thought to be responsible for many cases of neuropathic pain (pain related to dysfunction of the nerve tissues themselves) (9).

Most importantly for manual therapists, remember that you cannot rub nerve inflammation away. This is the key point to remember for effective work with sciatica (and other nerve pain). Since sciatic nerve inflammation is caused by pressure, applying more pressure will usually not help. With this in mind, it is typically best to

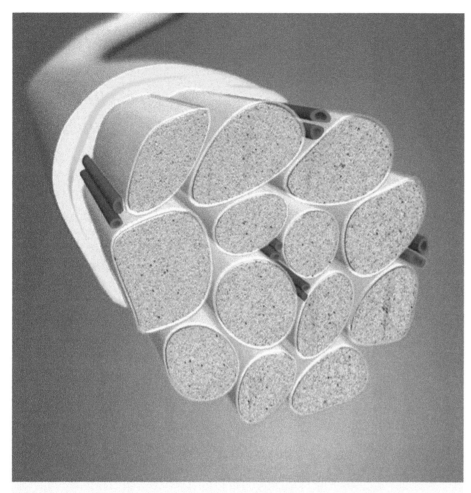

Figure 11.6

A peripheral nerve's connective tissue includes the inner perineurium (light tan), which encloses bundles of axons (dark beige) and the epineurium (green); and the outer wrapping of the nerve, which contains the nerve's internal blood supply (red and blue).

and foot. Like all peripheral nerves, these neurons are wrapped and bundled within various layers of connective tissue, the outermost layer being the epineurium (Figure 11.6), which is a continuation of the arachnoid and dural layers surrounding the central nervous system. The connective tissues of a nerve function to:

1. help maintain its internal electrochemical environment
2. carry the nerve's intrinsic blood vessels and sensory nerves

avoid exerting direct manual pressure on the sciatic nerve; instead, our goal is to increase "nerve glide": decompress the nerve's passageways, and release nerve sheaths from their adjoining structures to restore normal neural movement, freedom, and elastic sliding.

Sciatic Nerve Glide Test

Appendicular sciatica can be related to sciatic nerve entrapment at any of these sites:

- Under, over, through, or around the piriformis muscle or other external hip rotators (as discussed below)
- Between the quadratus femoris and gluteus maximus
- In the intermuscular septum between the biceps femoris and the adductor magnus in the posterior thigh.

These entrapment sites can be assessed with the Sciatic Glide Test. To perform the test, have your client lie supine with the hip and knee flexed on the affected side (Figure 11.7). Direct your client to actively straighten the bent knee of his or her raised leg (Figure 11.8). Extending just the knee from 90 degrees to fully straight stretches the sciatic nerve by about 1.5–2.5 inches; adding ankle dorsiflexion (as pictured) typically adds another half-inch of stretch (10). Thus, if straightening the affected leg increases sciatic symptoms, nerve tethering in the hip or leg is a likely contributor to the sciatic pain.

You can get even more specific about where to begin your work by asking your client to compare the sensations of straightening the affected and unaffected legs, and to direct you to any sites of increased pain or sensitivity. Nerve pain typically radiates distally, so the entrapment causing the pain resulting from this test is usually at the site of pain, or proximal to it[4] so it makes sense to start at the site of reported pain, and to work the nerve pathway proximally from there, retesting to track for any changes.

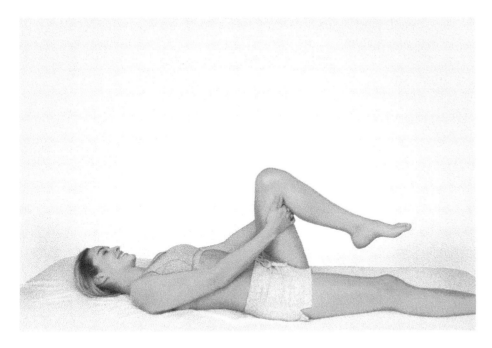

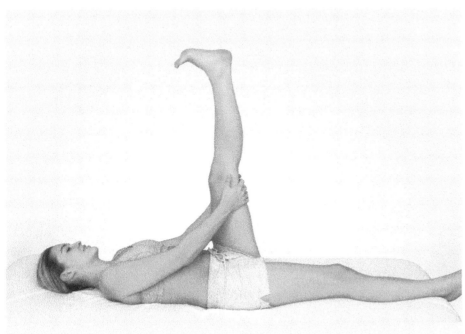

Figures 11.7/11.8

Given that the sciatic nerve stretches as much as 5 inches with lower-limb movements, the Sciatic Nerve Glide Test can help locate sciatic nerve entrapment sites. If knee extension and ankle dorsiflexion increase sciatic symptoms, nerve tethering in the hip or leg is likely, usually at the site of pain, or at a place proximal to it along the nerve's pathway.

4 As mentioned in the text, the entrapment site is usually at or proximal to the place where pain is felt by the client. However, referral patterns are common (typically involving gluteus maximus, medius, and minimus; rotators; or hamstrings), and like other referred pain, these are sometimes unpredictable and aren't easily explainable by direct neural connections.

Here are two variations to the Sciatic Nerve Glide Test (not pictured):

1. If the client experiences increased sciatic pain when bringing the straightened leg across the body (hip flexion and adduction with knee extension), this can indicate piriformis involvement.

2. Bending the knee of the passive leg and placing the sole on the table can help differentiate between lumbar and non-lumbar tethering. Since the knee-up position decreases lumbar extension, suspect tethering at the lumbars (axial sciatica) if raising the knee on the passive side decreases the Glide Test's sciatic pain. (Axial sciatica is discussed earlier in this chapter.)

Use what you learnt from performing the Sciatic Glide Test to choose where to work next. Myofascial techniques (such as those described below), as well as stretching the rotators, gluteus, or hamstrings, are often particularly effective ways to release the neural sheath adhesions or myofascial restrictions that you have discovered with the Sciatic Glide Test.

The Sciatic Glide Test itself can also be helpful as a take-home client exercise to mobilize a tethered nerve. Clients should be cautioned not to do too many repetitions at once, or to repeat the maneuver more than once per day, to avoid continually irritating an already inflamed sciatic nerve.

Other causes of appendicular sciatic pain

In addition to the soft-tissue impingements listed above, the following issues can also contribute to appendicular sciatic pain:

- Prolonged sitting, either from direct pressure on the sciatic nerve from wallets, bucket seats, etc.; or from postural strain resulting from hip flexion contracture or posterior pelvic rolling (slumping).

- Driving can increase leg tightness from pressing on the gas pedal, as well as from sitting (driving is also a risk factor for disc issues).
- Hypertrophy (overdevelopment and enlargement) of the piriformis, rotators, or hamstrings, especially when combined with repetitive motions (as in prolonged exercise).
- Structural and tissue changes associated with pregnancy and postpartum.
- Direct trauma to the sciatic nerve, tumors or infections, or scarring or thickening of adjacent soft tissues.

Some of the causes noted above suggest their own solutions, which often involve changes in activities or ergonomics. There are also many reports of appendicular sciatic relief being found in regular stretching (yoga's Pigeon Pose or Eka Pada Kapotasana, in particular), or from balanced strengthening and conditioning (strengthening the abductors, for example, can counterbalance and relieve hypertoned rotators and adductors).

Since appendicular sciatic entrapments are most often soft-tissue restrictions, these types of entrapments frequently respond quite well to focused and thorough hands-on myofascial work. I will describe hands-on techniques for working with the appendicular sciatic nerve entrapments, identified with the Sciatic Nerve Glide test.

Working with appendicular sciatica

A brief review of some important points: because axial sciatica can be associated with spinal instability (which can be worsened by indiscriminate deep work), the safest approach to this type of sciatica is easing the whole-body guarding and stress that accompany chronic pain, rather than performing deep, focused work on the lumbar nerve roots themselves. Persistent axial sciatic symptoms (as described above) can be a reason

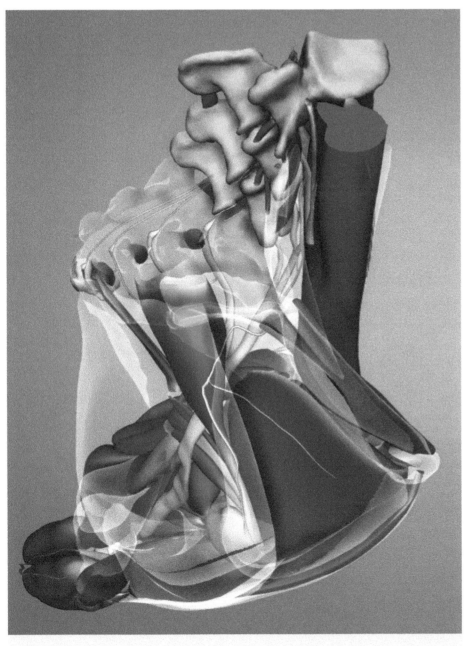

Figure 11.9

The sciatic nerve pathway, from above. Originating from spinal nerves L4–S3, which pass through and lie posterior to the psoas muscle, the sciatic nerve emerges from the pelvis and passes between the structures of the hip and posterior thigh. Impingement anywhere along its pathway can lead to the symptoms of sciatica.

for referral to a rehabilitation specialist, such as a physical therapist, chiropractor, or orthopedist.

By contrast, with appendicular sciatica, our approach is different. Appendicular sciatica is characterized by increased pain from sitting; stepping up stairs or inclines; from the direct pressure of sexual intercourse in women; or with resisted active external rotation of the femur. Appendicular sciatica can be just as painful as axial sciatica, but it is generally more amenable and responsive to soft-tissue work. This is because, in appendicular sciatica, it is usually soft tissue itself that entraps the sciatic nerve, as opposed to the bony or fibrocartilaginous entrapments that are typical in axial sciatica.

Our intention when working with appendicular sciatica is to facilitate normal nerve glide by releasing any tethering or compressing myofascial entrapments. These entrapment sites can often be identified using the Sciatic Nerve Glide Test described above. Here are three techniques that serve as examples of ways to safely and effectively ease the most common appendicular sciatic nerve entrapments:

Rotator (Piriformis) Technique

See video of the Rotators/Piriformis Technique at http:// advanced-trainings. com/v/pa10.html.

Sciatic nerve entrapment by the piriformis ("pear-shaped") muscle is probably the most common cause of appendicular sciatica. As mentioned earlier, the piriformis accounts for about 70 percent of all non-lumbar sciatic pain, according to one large-scale study (11). "Piriformis Syndrome" was first described in 1928, and its causes have been well studied and debated in the years since. It is also known as "pseudosciatica," or Type II Sciatica in chiropractic terminology. (In our trainings at Advanced-Trainings.com, we emphasize the broader term "appendicular sciatica", since piriformis-related entrapment is just one of several types of

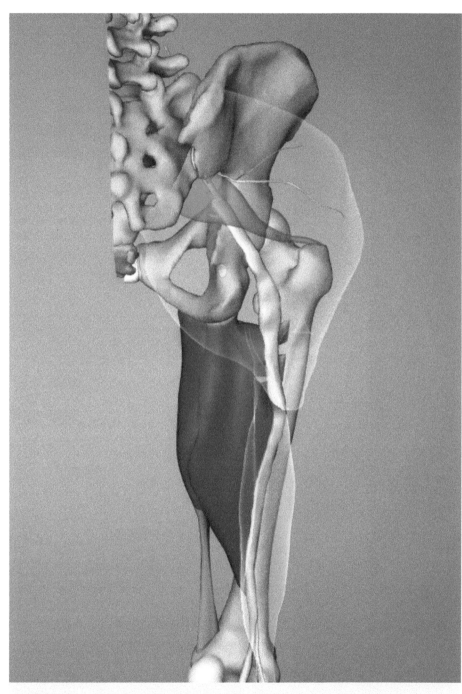

Figure 11.10

In appendicular sciatica, the sciatic nerve (yellow) can be entrapped by any of several structures in the hip or leg, including the piriformis (violet) and other rotators, or between the adductor magnus (red) and biceps femoris (green, transparent).

non-spinal sciatic nerve impingement.) Although sciatic symptoms are about equally common in men and women, piriformis syndrome occurs six times more frequently in women than in men (12), and some studies suggest that women's sciatica is often more severe (13). On the other hand, lumbar disc issues, which are often the cause of axial sciatica, are twice as common in men than women[5].

Anatomical variations in the sciatic nerve's pathway in relation to the piriformis have long been thought to be the cause of piriformis-related sciatic pain. In most people, the sciatic nerve passes deep to the piriformis (as it does in Figures 11.9 and 11.10), but 15 to 30 percent of people have variations in this arrangement (15) which can include:

- the nerve passing superficial to the piriformis;
- the nerve passing through the split belly of the muscle; and
- the split nerve passing in two parts around the piriformis.

However, some researchers question whether these anatomical variations have any significant bearing on sciatic symptoms, as they correlate poorly with actual sciatic symptoms (16). In a manual therapy setting, these variations are probably more interesting as anatomical trivia than as clinically useful information, since it is questionable whether variations in the piriformis/sciatic nerve arrangement – even if they were known – would change one's hands-on therapeutic approach. In other words, whatever the anatomy, the most practical strategy is usually to do some work and see how the symptoms respond, then adjust your approach accordingly.

Piriformis entrapment does not occur without reason or cause. Some of the other structural and functional factors that may trigger piriformis-related sciatic pain include:

- Internal rotation of the hip or leg, since during gait the piriformis may contract to counteract

---

5 "Males are affected approximately twice as often as females by lumbar disc issues, except in adolescents where there is a small female preponderance, probably due to earlier skeletal maturity. White-collar and professional employees are the least likely to be affected by lumbar disc herniations, and motor vehicle drivers are the most likely. The driver who spends greater than 50% of the working day behind the wheel has a three-fold increased risk, whereas the lorry [truck] driver has a five-fold increased risk." (14)

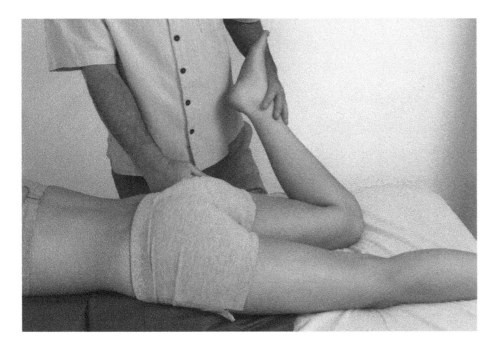

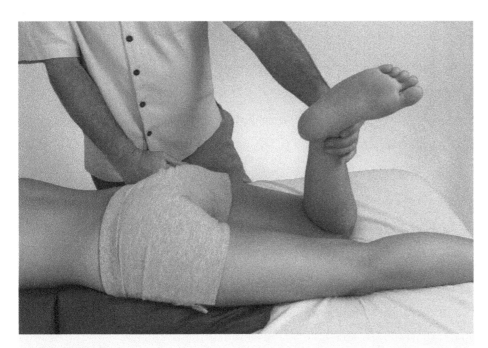

Figures 11.11 /11.12

The Rotator Technique: use static pressure on the piriformis attachments on the greater trochanter, combined with femur rotation.

tendencies towards internal rotation. Internal hip rotation, in turn, can be related to ankle pronation or myofascial imbalances (for example, tightness or fascial binding of the antero-lateral fascia lata, the medial hamstrings, or the posterior adductors).

- Sacral position and movement restrictions (since the piriformis acts on the sacrum), such as will be seen when there are sacroiliac joint issues, leg length differences, or ilia mobility imbalances.

Whatever the cause of piriformis entrapment, the Rotator Technique is an efficient and effective way to assess and release any local nerve impingement related to the piriformis, as well as the other external rotators (such as the quadratus femoris) that can have a bearing on sciatic nerve health.

To perform the technique, start with your client prone and the knee of the affected leg flexed. Use the lower leg to slowly roll the femur into internal and external rotation (Figures 11.11 and 11.12). With the soft fist of your other hand, gently apply firm, static pressure to various aspects of the greater trochanter, which is the distal attach-ment of the piriformis and other rotators. Use both hands; with the hand moving your client's leg, feel through the client's structure for the resistance of your static hand on the rotators.

Once you feel a change in the tissue's resilience, release the pressure, move your soft fist to another location, and slowly roll the femur again, feeling for restrictions in the new location. Be thorough; use this technique throughout the buttock and rotator region, but avoid putting direct pres-sure on the sciatic nerve itself. (The nerve runs midway between the trochanter and lateral edge of the sacrum, and pressure on it will be felt by your client as tenderness or an electric sensa-tion.) Rather than indiscriminately mashing the nerve and tissues here, imagine freeing the

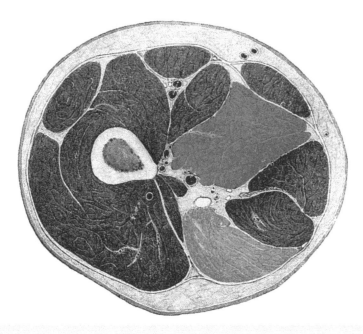

Figure 11.13

In the thigh, the sciatic nerve (yellow) lies within the thick connective tissue septum between the biceps femoris (green) and adductor magnus (orange).

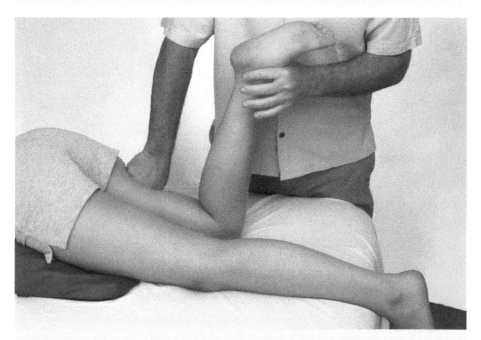

Figure 11.14

In the Biceps Femoris/Adductor Magnus Technique, passive femur rotation is used to roll these two structures apart, opening the nerve tract like a scroll.

Key points: Rotator (Piriformis) Technique

Indications include:
- Appendicular sciatic pain (see text).
- Positive (painful) Piriformis Test or Sciatic Glide Test
- Pain in superior gluteal nerve distribution area (upper gluteals; low back).

Purpose
- Assess and release any sciatic or superior gluteal nerve impingement related to the myofascial of the piriformis and/or other external hip rotators.

Instructions
- As you apply static pressure to the rotator attachments on the femur, use passive femoral rotation to slowly roll the greater trochanter under your static soft fist. Feel for tissue differentiation and elasticity change.

Cautions
- Avoid excessive or prolonged pressure directly on an inflamed sciatic nerve. Work tissues around the nerve, particularly their attachments, to increase tissue differentiation and elasticity.

nerve by releasing and separating any inelastic or adhered structures that surround it.

As its name suggests, the superior gluteal nerve is in the superior portion of this gluteal region (visible superior to the piriformis in Figures 11.9 and 11.10). Although considerably smaller than the sciatic nerve, it can be a source of sciatic-like pain in the upper buttock and lower back. If your client experiences pain here, you can use the Rotator Technique to release the tissues around this nerve as well.

Biceps Femoris/Adductor Magnus Technique

Distal to the rotators, the sciatic nerve can be impinged or tethered within the structures of the

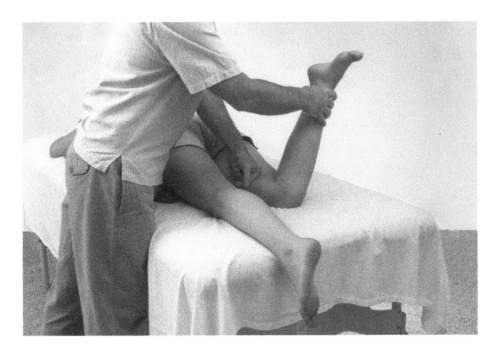

posterior thigh, particularly where it lies within the thick connective tissue of the intermuscular septum between the biceps femoris and adductor magnus (Figure 11.13) (17). We can adapt the Rotator Technique to help differentiate these powerful leg structures from one another, and in so doing, we can provide more freedom for the nerve. Begin with the biceps femoris, which is the most lateral of the hamstrings. As in the Rotator Technique, use gentle medial rotation of the femur with one hand, while the soft fist

---

Key points: Biceps Femoris/Adductor Magnus Technique

Indications:
- Appendicular sciatic pain (see text).
- Positive (painful) Sciatic Glide Test or Bowstring Test.
- Nerve pain in posterior thigh.

Purpose
- Assess and release any sciatic nerve impingement related to the intermuscular septum between biceps femoris and adductor magnus.

Instructions
- Anchor biceps femoris laterally as you use passive leg rotation to roll the adductor magnus medially. Feel for tissue differentiation at the intermuscular septum between adductor magnus and biceps femoris. Repeat with opposite placement (anchor adductor magnus medially, roll biceps femoris laterally).

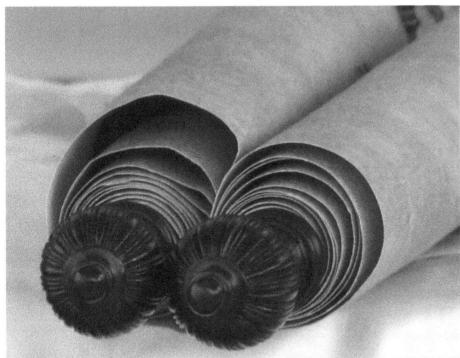

Figures 11.15/11.16

In the Biceps Femoris/Adductor Magnus Technique, passive femur rotation is used to roll these two structures apart, opening the nerve tract like a scroll.

of your other hand rolls the biceps laterally off the underlying femur and adductor magnus (Figure 11.14). At the comfortable extreme of the allowed motion, pause, wait, and feel for tissue release. Work the entire length of the biceps femoris, including its attachments on the ischial tuberosity. (If these attachments are particularly tender, as in "hamstring syndrome," use direct

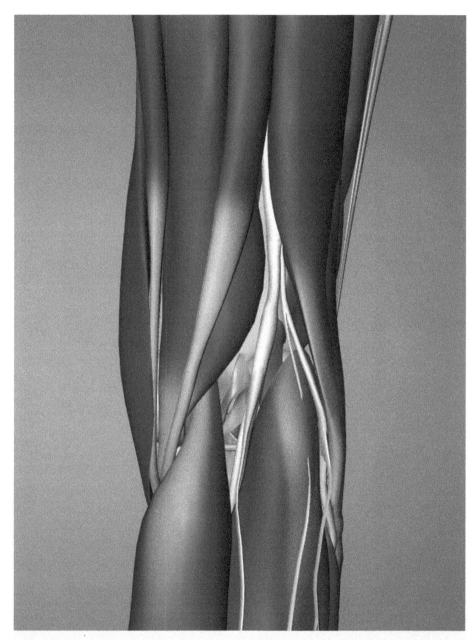

Figure 11.17

The sciatic nerve in the upper recesses of the popliteal space, where it emerges from between the medial and lateral hamstrings.

work on the irritated attachments cautiously, monitoring how your client responds in the days after the session.)

After laterally releasing the biceps femoris, move to the other side of the table and use lateral rotation of the femur to medially release the adductor magnus of the same leg (Figure 11.15). Imagine rolling the magnus and biceps away from one another like the two parts of a scroll (Figure 11.16), opening up the space between for the sciatic nerve.

Sciatic Traction Technique

Although in most cases it is advisable to avoid putting direct pressure on a nerve itself, sometimes distal traction (when carefully applied directly to the sciatic nerve) can free entrapments in the posterior thigh or hip that other techniques are not quite able to address.

Once the large muscles of the posterior leg have been differentiated with the previous techniques, perform the Sciatic Traction Technique by using the fingers of both hands to wrap around the knee into the popliteal space (behind the knee; Figures 11.18 and 11.19). The sciatic nerve is easily palpated in the upper recesses of the popliteal space, where it emerges between the medial and lateral hamstrings (Figure 11.17). The nerve will feel softer than the muscles and tendons that most soft-tissue therapists are accustomed to feeling for; in fact, most manual therapists subconsciously avoid the nerves, so for many practitioners, looking for the nerve will require a change of approach. A healthy sciatic nerve has the consistency and size of a large earthworm or a thick, al dente linguini noodle. An irritated nerve will often be harder or stringier (and thus easier to palpate). Until you are practiced at finding the sciatic nerve here, your client's moment-by-moment

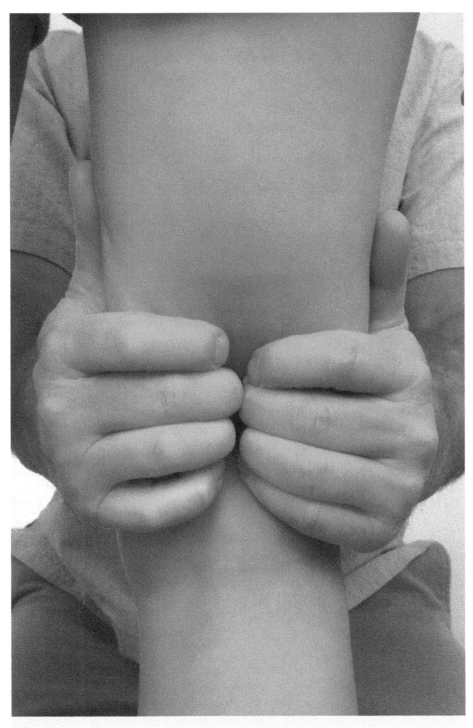

Figure 11.18

The Sciatic Traction Technique. Use gentle pressure to feel for and distally stretch any sciatic nerve connective tissue tethering in the posterior thigh. Use your client's feedback to help comfortably locate the nerve.

report will be your most reliable guide – when you find the nerve, it will cause a mild tingling or electric sensation. The more the nerve is irritated in this region, the more sensitive it will be, so begin slowly to avoid unnecessary aggravation.

Once you have located the nerve, apply gentle traction to it as your client slowly lifts his or her knee slightly (Figure 11.19). This will allow you to pull the nerve distally, freeing its lower section as it passes between the hamstrings. When done correctly with a client who has sciatic impingement here, this technique can yield a sense of immediate relief.

Here and elsewhere, however, it is good to keep in mind that relief from sciatic pain does not always come right away. Even when you have thoroughly released the connective tissue tethering that irritates a nerve, the inflammation

Key points: Sciatic Traction Technique

Indications
- Appendicular sciatic pain (see text).
- Positive (painful) Sciatic Glide Test or Bowstring test.

Purpose
- Assess and release any sciatic nerve impingement related to reduced nerve glide in hip or posterior thigh.

Instructions
- After preparing the posterior thigh with other work, apply gentle distal traction to the sciatic nerve at the popliteal space, as client slowly lifts the knee (slight hip flexion). Feel for glide of the nerve within its surrounding fasciae.

Movements
- Slow active hip flexion.

Cautions
- Limit the duration and intensity of your work to avoid aggravating an inflamed sciatic nerve.

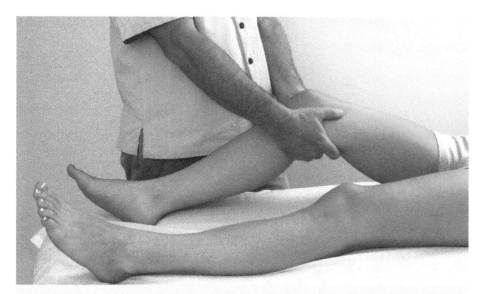

Figure 11.19

The Sciatic Traction Technique. Continue to apply gentle traction to the sciatic nerve sheath, as your client slowly lifts his or her knee.

can take time to subside. In some cases, long-term neuropathic pain (of which sciatic pain is one kind) can lead to changes in nerve function that takes time to reverse. The non-noxious tactile stimulation of your work is therapeutic in these cases, so remember that you are helping the nerve to recover its normal function by just doing your work.

In most cases, plan to address sciatica over a series of sessions, and make sure that your client is aware that habitual activity modification, stretching, or exercise may be necessary to augment your hands-on work. Be sure to refer stubborn cases for medical or orthopedic examination, especially if you suspect lumbar involvement. Even if the nerve entrapment is released in a single session (which does happen), an inflamed nerve can take time to heal, so be patient, thorough and, as always, do not hesitate to seek supervision or advice.

References

[1] Konstantinou, K. and Dunn, K.M. (2008) Sciatica: review of epidemiological studies and prevalence estimates. *Spine*. Oct 15, 33(22):p. 2464–72.

[2] Konstantinou, K. (2008) ibid.

[3] Valat, J.P. et al. (2010) Sciatica: Best Practices. *Res Clinical Rheumatology*. Apr; 24(2). p. 241–52.

[4] As mentioned by Jim Donak and Tom Myers in an Aug 2010 discussion at http://www.facebook.com/topic.php?uid=120301201315055&topic=181 [accessed April 2014]

[5] Bogduk, N. (2005) *Clinical anatomy of the lumber spine and sacrum* (4th ed). Churchill Livingston.

[6] Devillé, W.L. et al. (2000) The test of Lasègue: Systematic review of the accuracy in diagnosing herniated discs. *Spine*. 25(9). p. 1140–7.

[7] Filler, A., Haynes, J., Jordan, S. et al. (2005) Sciatica of nondisc origin and piriformis syndrome: diagnosis by magnetic resonance neurography and interventional magnetic resonance imaging with outcome study of resulting treatment. *Journal of Neurosurgery*: Spine. 2(2). p. 99–115.

[8] Belth, I.D. et al. An assessment of the adaptive mechanisms within and surrounding the peripheral nervous system, during changes in nerve bed length resulting from underlying joint movement. From: *Moving in on Pain: Conference Proceedings*. April 1995 Butterworth-Heinemann; 1st edition (December 27, 1995) p. 194–196.

[9] Asbury, A.K. and Fields, H.L. (1984) Pain due to peripheral nerve damage: an hypothesis. *Neurology*. 34. p. 1587–1590.

[10] Belth, I.D. et al. Ibid.

[11] Filler, A., Haynes, J., Jordan, S. et al. (2005) Journal of Neurosurgery: *Spine*. 2(2). p. 99–115.

[12] Otis, C. http://www.sportsdoctor.com/articles/sciatica3.html. [accessed April 2014]

[13] Swierzewski, S.J. (reviewer). Sciatica Overview, Incidence and Prevalence of Sciatica. http://www.healthcommunities.com/sciatica/sciatica-overview.shtml. [accessed April 2014]

[14] Noordeen, Hilali et al. (2009) *Interactive Spine* v1.66. Primal Pictures Ltd.

[15] Pokorný, D. et al (2006). Topographic variations of the relationship of the sciatic nerve and the piriformis muscle and its relevance to palsy after total hip arthroplasty. *Surg Radiol Anat*. 28(1). p. 88–91.

[16] Benzon, H.T. et al (2003). Piriformis syndrome: anatomic considerations, a new injection technique, and a review of the literature. *Anesthesiology*. 98(6) p. 1442–8.

[17] Saikku, K. et al. (2010) Entrapment of the proximal sciatic nerve by the hamstring tendons. *Acta Orthop. Belg*. 76. p. 321–324.

Picture credits

Study Guide

Sciatic Pain

1 **Why does the text say that it is useful to distinguish axial from appendicular sciatica?**

a manual therapy does not generally help axial sciatica
b manual therapy does not generally help appendicular sciatica
c knowing the type can help determine where to work
d appendicular sciatica should be referred to a specialist

2 **According to this chapter, when would referring your client with sciatic pain to a specialist be indicated?**

a symptoms increase with sitting
b symptoms do not change with the SLT
c symptoms are persistent or severe
d symptoms increase during the piriformis test

3 **Which of these signs is NOT typical of axial sciatica (unless accompanied by appendicular sciatica)?**

a sciatic scoliosis (leaning)
b positive (painful) SLT
c positive (painful) piriformis test
d pain in the lower back (along with gluteal and/or hip pain)

4 **The text states that from the site of entrapment, nerve pain typically radiates:**

a proximally
b distally
c medially
d laterally

5 **The text states that in normal movement, an adult's sciatic nerve typically stretches:**

a 0.3 to 0.5 mm
b 3 to 5 mm
c 0.3 to 0.5 inches
d 3 to 5 inches

For Answer Keys, visit www.Advanced-Trainings.com/v1key/

The Sacrotuberous Ligament

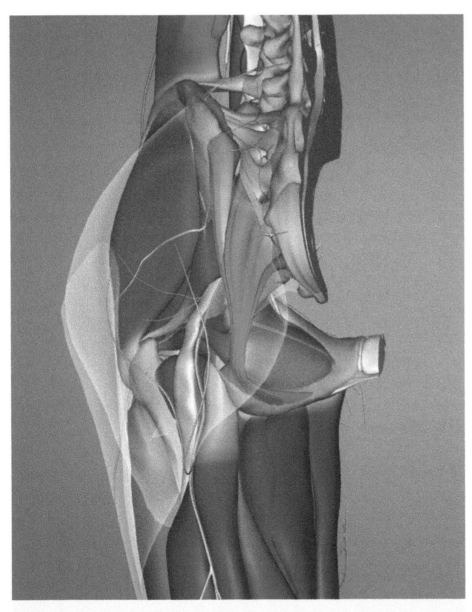

Figure 12.1

The sacrotuberous ligament (orange) is involved in conditions as varied as low back pain, sciatica (the sciatic nerve is the large yellow structure lateral to the sacrotuberous ligament), sacroiliac joint pain (the sacroiliac ligament is green), hamstring syndrome, postural issues, and more. The falciform process (purple) is indicated in perineal pain and numbness, as the pudendal nerve can become entrapped here.

The sacrotuberous ligaments lie at a crucial structural crossroads in the human body. As mediators between the spine and legs, this pair of strong, broad ligaments bridges the upper and lower body (Figure 12.1). As stabilizers of the sacrum, they accommodate the left/right forces of foot-to-foot weight transfer. And, in efficient walking and running, these ligaments are key connective tissue links in the chain of kinetic energy uptake, adding spring to each step (1).

That is, they do these things when they're balanced and healthy. When they aren't, the sacrotuberous ligaments can play an equally significant role in many client complaints, including low back pain, a condition that in the USA affects almost 90 percent of all people at some point in their lives (2). While the sacrotuberous ligament isn't involved in all types of back pain, a very large portion of low back pain cases stem from issues related to these important ligaments, such as lumbar curvature and strain, sacral angle and tilt, sacroiliac joint health, and more, making the sacrotuberous ligaments crucial structures to address whenever clients complain of lumbar pain.

In addition to low back pain, working with the sacrotuberous ligaments is an important part of addressing many other conditions, such as:

- Sacroiliac joint hypermobility, hypomobility, and pain. When one sacrotuberous ligament is tighter than the other, the sacrotuberous ligaments are associated with sacral rotation, side-bending, or fixation
- Coccyx (tailbone) injuries and pain, since the sacrotuberous ligament attaches to and stabilizes the coccyx
- Sciatic pain (both axial and appendicular), including piriformis syndrome, since the sciatic nerve and piriformis are close neighbors

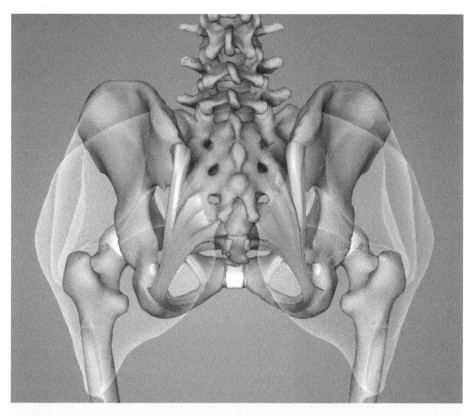

Figure 12.2

The bilateral arrangement of the sacrotuberous ligaments gives them a key role in stabilizing the sacrum against torquing and tilting. The sacrotuberous ligaments can be strained or injured by activities involving twisting or arching the low back; asymmetries will also result from functional issues habit and posture) or structural issues (such as leg length difference).

- Peroneal pain and numbness, as the pudendal or cutaneous nerves can become entrapped within the sacrotuberous ligament, or between it and the sacrospinous ligaments
- Painful sitting, hamstring tendonitis, or ischial bursitis
- Leg length differences, both anatomical and functional
- Spinal scoliosis or lordosis (swayback)
- Pelvic torsions, upslip, and pubic symphysis irritation
- Slumped or twisted posture in sitting or standing, since the sacrotuberous ligaments are key determinants of sacral angle and the resulting segmental relationships all the way through the body
- Pelvic floor, prostate, and urogenital issues, because muscles and fascias of these structures attach to the sacrotuberous ligaments.

In addition, many models of movement and fascial continuity describe the sacrotuberous ligament as a key structure. At its superior origin at the PSIS (Figure 12.2), its fibers are continuous with the deep fascia of the lumbar intermuscular aponeurosis (3); inferiorly, its superficial fibers cross the ischial tuberosity in about 50 percent of people, and are thus continuous with the biceps femoris tendon in the leg (4). Each of these structures continues in turn as parts of longer chains. These long connections through the body lend the sacrotuberous ligament (in its central location) its linchpin role in whole-body theories of connective tissue relationships, such as Thomas Myers' Anatomy Trains model, the ipsilateral longitudinal sling concept in functional medicine, or Gracovetsky's Spinal Engine theory.

Functionally, the bilaterally oblique arrangement of the two sacrotuberous ligaments serves to prevent the sacrum from being tipped forward (into anterior nutation) by the downward pressure of the spine. Together with the sacroiliac and sacrospinous ligaments, the sacrotuberous ligaments also stabilize the sacrum against excessive sidebending and twisting within the pelvis. Because of this paired, left-right arrangement, a side-to-side imbalance in the sacrotuberous ligaments' length or tension will be linked to sacral rotation, pelvic torsion, and strain on the SI joints and low back.

Sorting out the root cause of sacrotuberous ligament imbalances can be a chicken-or-egg pursuit: are the ligaments different left and right because of a pelvic torsion, or is their difference causing the pelvis asymmetry? Often, determining cause can be elusive. On the other hand, an injury or an observable structural irregularity (such as an anatomical leg length difference) can make the root cause of a ligament imbalance clearer. The sacrotuberous ligament can be strained or injured in sports and activities that involve arching or twisting the low back, such as basketball, tennis, golfing, gymnastics, hurdles or jumping, pitching, or volleyball spiking. Falls onto the buttocks or other direct trauma can strain or tear the sacrotuberous ligament, as well as injure the coccyx. Lifting or bending injuries, repetitive and asymmetrical activities, hamstring tendonitis, and pregnancy can all cause sacrotuberous ligament strain and sensitivity as well. The result of any of these impairments is often inflammation, scarring, adhesions, pain, and loss of connective tissue adaptability.

Sacral balance

Even when the cause or source of a left/right sacrotuberous ligament imbalance is not apparent, such as when there isn't a clear mechanism of injury, your work here can nevertheless be helpful in addressing the sacrotuberous ligament-related conditions listed above.

Together with the sacroiliac and sacrospinous ligaments, the sacrotuberous ligaments stabilize the sacrum and pelvis against excessive sidebending and twisting. The bony space between the sacrum and the ischial tuberosity is often palpably different left to right, with one side often being more open or wider than the other; this indicates an asymmetrical pelvic pattern, most likely involving sacral sidebend or rotation. Sacral biomechanics are complex and quite arcane, and their details are beyond the scope of this chapter. However, one very useful principle is that if the space between two bones (the sacrum and the ischial tuberosity, in this example) is shorter on one side of the body, the ligament on the shorter side will be tighter or harder if it is a contributor to the asymmetry, but softer if it is being slackened by the bony asymmetry (that is, if the asymmetry is due to other forces or structures, and not the ligament itself). Furthermore, if a ligament is tighter on the longer or wider side, is it most likely being stretched by the structural asymmetry, and the root cause lies elsewhere (for example, leg length, patterns of usage, etc.).

Using these principles, you would then work more with the tighter or harder sacrotuberous ligament if it was on the side of the sacrum with less space between it and the ischial tuberosity (the shorter or narrower side), but work elsewhere in the body (such as the hamstrings or hip joint) when the tighter sacrotuberous ligament is on the longer side.

If you suspect sacrotuberous ligament involvement in your client's symptoms, but don't perceive a length or tissue difference left and right, let your client's experience be your guide: work one side, and then have your client get up and walk or bend. Is that easier or less painful than before? You're on track. Not easier? Work the other side's sacrotuberous ligament, and recheck. Clients will frequently report less pain and greater ease when you work in this way to balance any left/right differences you find in the sacrotuberous ligaments.

See video of the Sacrotuberous Ligament Technique at http://advanced-trainings.com/v/pa11.html.

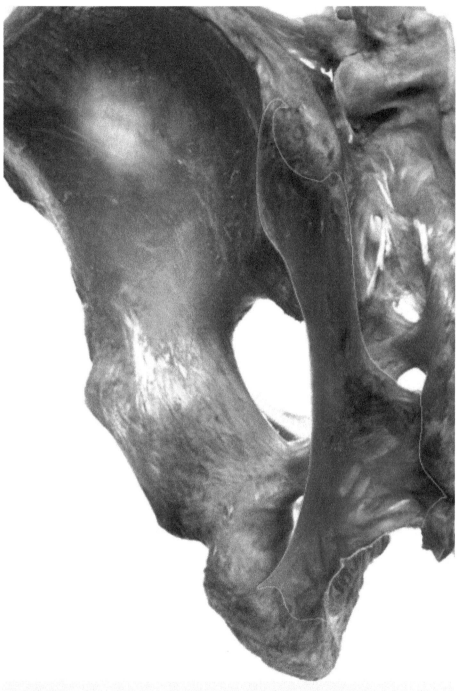

Figure 12.3

The sacrotuberous ligament (orange) spans the distance between the PSIS at its upper end, along the lateral side of the sacrum and coccyx, to the ischial tuberosity inferiorly. Comparing left- and right-side differences in the bony space lateral to the sacrum and coccyx can give clues to imbalances in the sacrotuberous ligaments.

Sacrotuberous Ligament Technique

Because the ligaments are in a personal or private part of the body, before working with the sacrotuberous ligaments, it is important to get your client's explicit consent and buy-in. Inform your client of the reasons for working the ligaments. I will often show my clients the anatomy involved, and I always explain why I think work here might be helpful by relating it to their particular symptoms. If you haven't already been trained in sacrotuberous ligament work, get familiar with the anatomy of the area by practicing palpation with a colleague or learning partner, before attempting these techniques on a client.

Once you have your client's permission to work their sacrotuberous ligaments, stand at his or her side, and begin by making tactile contact somewhere other than the ligament itself (such as the knee or low back). In other words, ease into the area being worked. Checking in with your client all the while, reach across the body to find the opposite side ischial tuberosity with one hand, and the posterior (back) side of the coccyx with the other. The sacrotuberous ligament runs between these two landmarks, just anterior (deep) to the medial margin of gluteus maximus. Palpate the sacrotuberous ligament on the lateral side of the upper gluteal cleft (Figure 12.7). Work on the opposite side from where you're standing, as this gives a better angle for your thumbs to gently but firmly press into the ligament's inferomedial margin (Figures 12.4 and 12.5). You aren't trying to feel the ligament through the gluteus; rather, you're feeling in front of (anterior to) the gluteus maximus. The ligament will feel ropy or hard on most people; remember, it is in front of (deep or anterior to) the gluteal mound.

Keep your thumbs together in order to avoid straining them. Switch sides of the table and use this stable "mono-thumb" to compare the hardness and tension of the left and right ligaments. Also compare the bony space and tissue

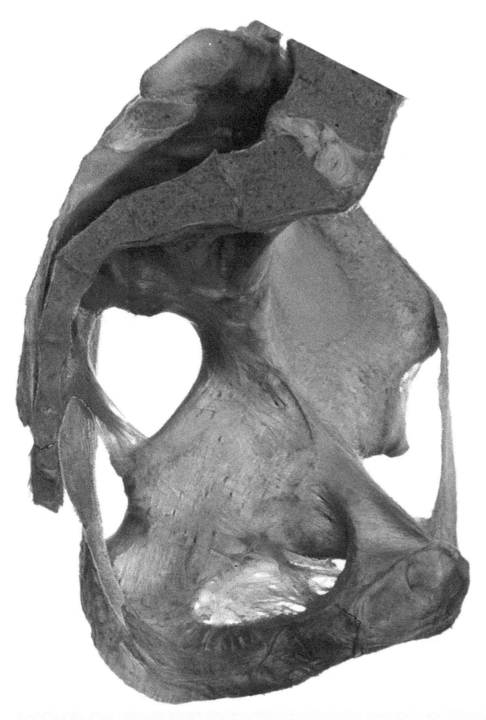

quality on each side of the coccyx (Figure 12.3). The sacrotuberous ligament and sacrospinous ligaments converge here, and both can contribute to coccyx pain or misalignment.

Once you've assessed both sides, spend comparatively more time on the side where you found the harder ligament, together with less bony space. Beginning with the upper or proximal end of the ligament, find a level of pressure that your client can relax into, and wait for a sense of tissue release in each place before moving slightly to the next part of the ligament. Avoid sliding or friction – static, focused, firm but receptive touch will allow your client to release the tissues in a way that won't be possible if your touch is active or moving.

Around the coccyx itself, work patiently to gradually release the ligaments and tissues

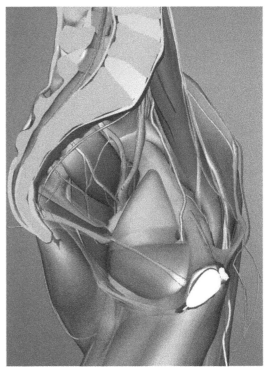

Figures 12.4/12.5

The sacrotuberous ligament (orange) viewed medially. Note its span along the ischial tuberosity and pubic ramus, and its position anterior (deep to) the gluteus maximus.

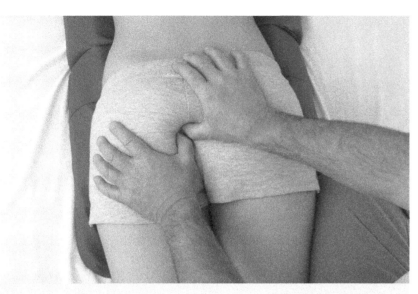

Figure 12.6

The Sacrotuberous Ligament Technique. Once you have your client's permission, assess the bony space and tissue tone on either side of the sacrum and coccyx.

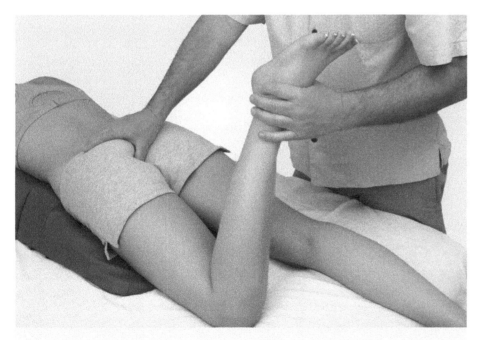

Figure 12.7

The Sacrotuberous Ligament Technique (continued). Use passive motion to release the sacrotuberous ligament on the shorter and tighter side.

surrounding the tailbone with sensitive, stationary thumb pressure. Again, spend more time on the shorter, harder, or narrower side of the coccyx. Rather than attempting to straighten any bony crookedness you find in the coccyx, your goal is evenness of tissue tone on each side of the tailbone, along with gentle desensitization of any painful or excessively guarded areas. If the coccyx has been injured, for example in a fall or in childbirth, it can be extremely sensitive. If you work slowly enough that your client can continue to relax and breathe freely, you'll see any hypersensitivity diminish.

After working the upper end of the sacrotuberous ligament, continue working up the length of each ligament, one area at a time. If there is perineal pain or numbness, pay special attention to the midsection of the sacrotuberous ligament, since it is here that the pudendal nerve can be entrapped between the sacrotuberous ligament and the deeper sacrospinous ligament. Continue your step-by-step release until you reach the ischial tuberosity. Alternatively, you can add passive or active leg rotation to access different aspects of the ligament (Figure 12.7). Another alternative is to work the sacrotuberous ligament with your client in a side lying or lateral recumbent position, carefully using the elbow to address the ligament on the lower side of the body (not pictured).

Key points: Sacrotuberous Ligament Technique

Indications include:
- Pelvic, coccyx, pubis, sacroiliac, low back, or sciatic pain;
- Perineal pain and numbness;
- Painful sitting, hamstring tendonitis, or ischial bursitis;
- Pain or mobility issues associated with asymmetrical patterns (scoliosis, pelvic asymmetries, leg length differences);
- Slumped, lordotic, or asymmetrical posture.

Purpose
- Balance any left/right differences in sacrotuberous resilience and span
- Differentiate ligaments from any inelastic adjacent tissues.

Instructions
- Using both thumbs together to avoid strain, work across the body to compare left and right:
  a) distance between sacrum and ischial tuberosity; and
  b) elasticity and density of sacrotuberous ligaments.
- Work hard/tighter ligament if on shorter side. (If on longer side, look elsewhere for cause of ligament strain, see text.)
- Work entire length of ligament, differentiating any inelastic tissues adjacent to ligaments.

Cautions
- Explain purpose for work beforehand and get explicit permission for working in this personal region.

Summary
To review our main points:
1. Work with the sacrotuberous ligaments to ease tissue restrictions around them, and to balance left/right asymmetries.
2. Practice on a peer first.
3. Be sensitive and thorough.
4. Stay in close verbal contact with your client as you work.

Finish your sacrotuberous ligament work on each side with special attention to the medial aspects of the tuberosities and ischial ramus, where pudendal nerve impingements can also occur in the area of the ligament's falciform ("crescent-shaped") process (Figure 12.1) [1.]

Done sensitively and properly, this work will feel deep and very effective, rather than invasive or overly personal. Including the sacrotuberous ligaments in your work will help you more effectively address a wide variety of structural and functional conditions, reflecting the critical role these structures play in efficient posture and function.

References

[1] Gracovetsky, S. (1988) *The Spinal Engine*. New York: Springer-Verlag.

[2] van Wingerden, J.P., Vleeming, A., Snijders, C.J. and Stoeckart, R. (1992) The spine-pelvis-leg mechanism; with a study of the sacrotuberous ligament. In: *Low back pain and its relation to the sacroiliac joint*. First Interdisciplinary World Congress on Low Back Pain and its relation to the Sacroiliac Joint. p.147–148, San Diego. Rotterdam: ECO. ISBN 90-9005121-X.

[3] Hammer, W. (2007) *Functional Soft-Tissue Examination and Treatment by Manual Methods*. Jones & Bartlett Learning. 438.

[4] Vleeming, A., Stoeckart, R. et al. (1989). The sacrotuberous ligament: a conceptual approach to its dynamic role in stabilizing the sacroiliac joint. *Clinical Biomechanics*. 4(4): p. 200–203.

Picture credits

Figures 12.1–12.5 courtesy Primal Pictures, used by permission.
Figures 12.6 and 12.7 courtesy Advanced-Trainings.com.

---

1 The falciform process of the sacrotuberous ligament, present on about five people in six, blends with the fascial sheath of the internal pudendal vessels and nerves.

Study Guide

The Sacrotuberous Ligament

1 As mentioned in the writing, how does the sacrotuberous ligament prevent anterior nutation of the sacrum?

a by its unilateral horizontal fiber arrangement
b by its connection to the hamstrings in some people
c by its bilateral oblique fiber arrangement
d by its impingement of the sciatic nerve

2 According to the text, what bony space is compared left and right to assess pelvic asymmetry and possible STL involvement?

a between the PSIS and the ischial tuberosity
b between the sacrum and the ischial tuberosity
c between the femur and the ischial tuberosity
d between the PSIS and the sacrum

3 Where does the writing recommend working if the bony space mentioned in question 2 is smaller on one side, and the sacrotuberous ligament feels tighter on that same side?

a the gluteals, hamstrings or low back
b the opposite side sacrotuberous ligament
c the opposite side coccyx or obturator internus
d the same side sacrotuberous ligament

4 What does the chapter state is important to get from the client before working their sacrotuberous ligament?

a a complete health history
b their current pain levels
c their explicit permission
d their goals for the session

5 As mentioned in the writing, which nerve can become entrapped between the sacrotuberous ligament and the sacrospinous ligament?

a pudendal
b sciatic
c peroneal
d superior gluteal

For Answer Keys, visit www.Advanced-Trainings.com/v1key/

The Sacroiliac Joints

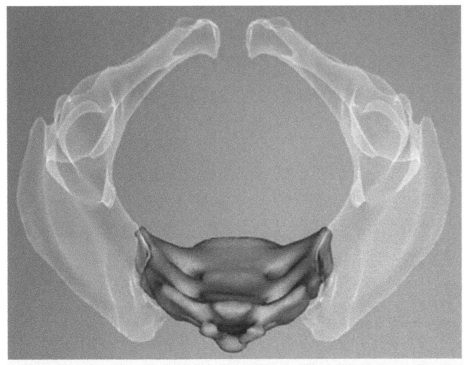

Figure 13.1

The sacroiliac joints are the articulation of the sacrum (opaque) with the hip bones (transparent). These important joints can be painful when they are either too loose or too tight. Hip, groin, sciatic, buttock or low back pain can result.

The sacroiliac joints (SIJs) are the body's meeting place. Here, the spine meets the pelvis, the upper body meets the lower body, the axial meets the appendicular skeleton, and the left and right sides meet the center. These deep, complex, and large articulations play a key role in walking, stepping, sitting, bending, and many other daily activities.

What is more, when there is SIJ pain, it can seem to affect the very core of our subjective experience, giving a sense of instability and disruption that, for many people, is reflected in their mood and outlook, as well as in their objective physical functioning.

Work with the sacroiliac joints (Figure 13.1) is indicated when clients experience any of the following:

- Low back pain, especially when unilateral (discussed below)
- Sciatic pain, both axial and appendicular (see Chapter 11, *Sciatic Pain*)
- Pain or sensitivity in the SIJs themselves, such as in sacroiliitis (inflamed joints) or sacroiliac (SI) dysfunction syndrome (too much or too little movement, also discussed below).

SI mobility and balance is also important whenever working with symptoms associated with asymmetrical patterns such as scoliosis, leg length discrepancies, asymmetrical activities and habits (for example, throwing sports or crossing one's legs), and other structural or functional patterns that demand extra accommodation at the sacral meeting place.

In this chapter, I will describe two gentle yet effective SIJ techniques. In addition to being useful in addressing the symptoms listed above, these two examples of SIJ techniques are effective ways to either:

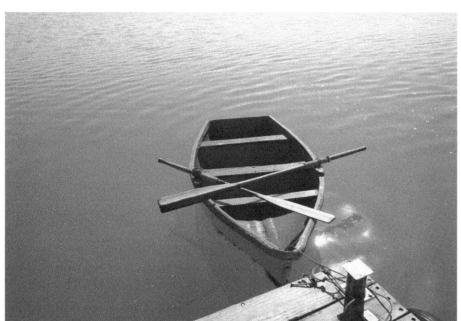

See video of the SI Anterior/Posterior Release Technique at http://advanced-trainings.com/v/pd03.html.

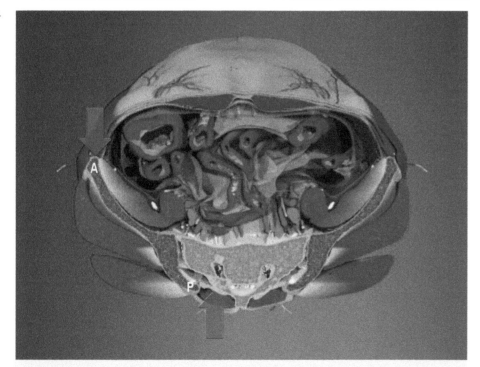

Figures 13.2/13.3

The sacrum (green) meets the ilium obliquely, so that anterior pressure on the sacrum will distract the SI joint. Purple arrows show hand placement for the SI Anterior/Posterior Release technique on the ASIS (A) and medial to PSIS (P). Feel through the sacral multifides, and wait for the sacrum to drift, analogous to pushing a boat away from a dock.

- Begin a session, since they tend to evoke a palliative parasympathetic response (the sacrum being one of the body's main locations for parasympathetic nerve ganglia)
- End a session, both because of their calming and quieting effect, and because ensuring sacral adaptability after working elsewhere is thought to aid in integration and help prevent post-session discomfort. (Ida P. Rolf, the originator of Rolfing Structural Integration, used sacral work as part of the closing ritual in most, if not all, of her sessions.)

SI Anterior/Posterior Release Technique

When SI motion is excessive, such as after an injury, the joints can become irritated. However, in walking and bending, there is a surprising amount of movement in healthy SIJs – they twist, glide, shear, and gap to a palpable degree. These are crucial for shock absorption, structural adaptability, and kinetic loading.

Since the planes of the SIJs are oblique (Figure 13.3), anterior to posterior movement of the sacrum in relation to the ilia will slightly distract (or open) the SIJ. We can use this principle to assess and release mobility restrictions at the SIJs.

With your client supine, begin by locating the posterior superior iliac spine (PSIS) on one side (Figures 13.4 and 13.5). Move your fingertips just medial to the PSIS, but stay lateral to the body's midline. You will be in a position to lift the sacrum anteriorly on that side. Slowly but firmly, lift with your fingertips. Maintain some flexion at each finger joint, leaving your wrist and arm as relaxed as possible to protect your forearm from any strain. Feel through the sacral multifides and erectors to sense the bony feel of the sacrum itself. Lift firmly and steadily, but gently.

Lightly rest your other hand on the same side's anterior superior iliac spine (ASIS) in order to encourage that ilium to drop posteriorly.

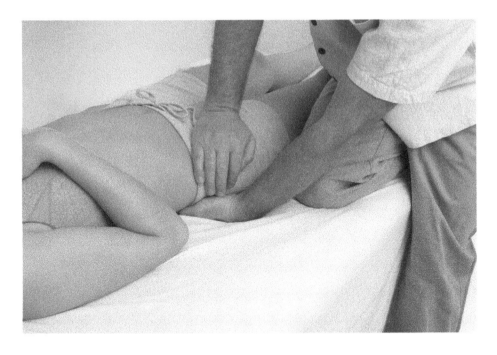

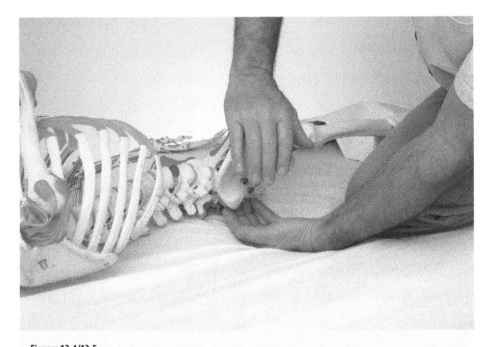

Figures 13.4/13.5

The SI Anterior/Posterior Release. Reach around the PSIS to lift the sacrum from below. The top hand on the ASIS is very light, encouraging the ilium to drop posteriorly and so gently distract (open) the SI joint space.

This anterior hand is much gentler and more receptive than the directive touch of the posterior hand. Since the pelvic girdle is built to transmit the force of gravity from the spine to the legs, it will respond to overt force from your hands by stiffening and stabilizing. Proceed slowly and lightly enough so that you do not evoke this stabilizing response. Although it may feel like you are using too little pressure to have an effect, if you are patient enough, the client's felt experience can be dramatic.

Use both hands to "listen" for a slight posterior yielding of the ilium and/or an anterior drifting of the sacrum. Although the amount of movement at the SIJ that can be considered normal is a subject of ongoing debate, computed tomography scans have shown 4–8 millimeters of PSIS motion here, even in the elderly (1). Thus, even though it is likely to be small, this movement will be quite tangible to both you and your client. Imagine pushing a large boat away from a dock (Figure 13.2). At first there appears to be nothing happening, but then slight movement becomes apparent after a few moments. The key is to wait for the release – it often takes 3–6 breaths to feel the drift happen; then, believe it when you feel it. Clients report sensations such as warmth spreading down their limb, or an overall softening of the pelvis, or an easing of the lower back. If clients report pain, it is likely a sign of joint irritation. If this is the case, ease off on the pressure you're using, finding the client's level of comfortable tolerance.

This technique is both an assessment and a release, so you can use it to compare and balance the left and right SIJs. SI stiffness is highly variable between individuals, but it has been shown to be more even side-to-side in asymptomatic individuals (2). If one side of the sacrum is particularly stiff or slow to respond, you can use the SI Wedge Technique (described next) to get a more specific release.

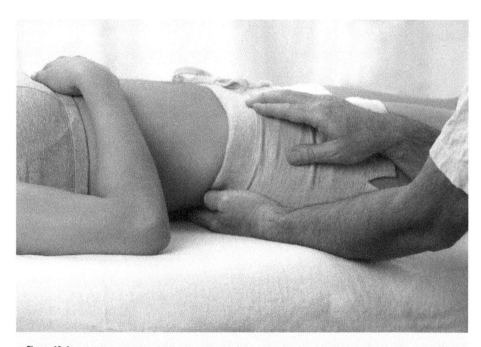

Figure 13.6

The Sacroiliac Wedge Technique.

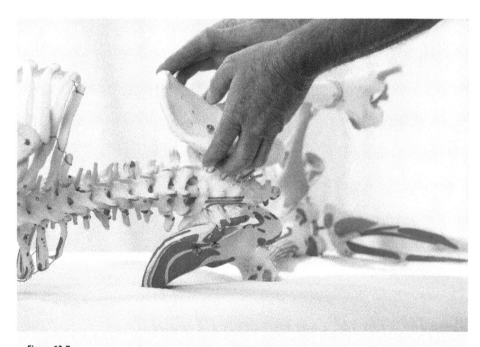

Figure 13.7

Hand positions for the Sacroiliac Wedge Technique: just medial to PSIS, and resting lightly on the ASIS.

Key points: SI Anterior/Posterior Release Technique

Indications include:
- Sacroiliac, low back, or sciatic pain.
- Pain or mobility issues associated with asymmetrical patterns (scoliosis, pelvic asymmetries, leg length differences).
- Preparation for or integration of other work.

Purpose
- Balance any left/right differences in anterior/posterior sacroiliac adaptability (both amplitude and quality of motion).
- Joint hydration and proprioceptive stimulation.
- Calming and quieting (via parasympathetic nervous system responses).

Instructions
- Assess SIJ A/P mobility by lifting one side of the sacrum anteriorly, while gently encouraging same-side innominate to drop posteriorly. Compare this to the opposite side's mobility.
- On the less mobile side, wait with static pressure for a slight yielding or drifting of the sacrum or innominate.

Sacroiliac Wedge Technique

As with the previous technique, the SI Wedge Technique can help reestablish normal mobility in a restricted SIJ. Try this variation when you find a restriction that does not seem to respond to the SI A/P Release Technique, or whenever you want a more specific release right at the SIJ.

Use the PSIS as a starting place – but instead of moving medially onto the sacrum, as we did in the previous technique – curl your fingers around the medial aspect of the PSIS. Like the last technique, this one involves lifting with the fingertips from underneath; however, rather than lifting the sacrum itself, stay close to the ilia, and lift into the SIJ space in a laterally oblique direction (Figures 13.6, 13.7, and 13.8).

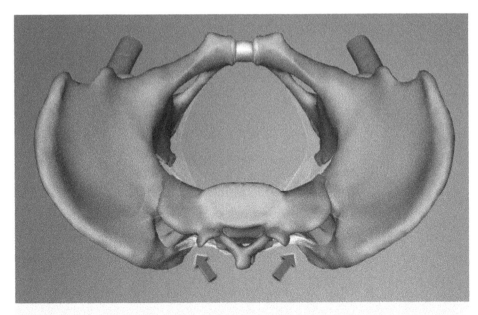

Figure 13.8

The Sacroiliac Wedge Technique. Lift with fingertips just medially to the PSIS to form a gentle wedge (arrows) into the SI joint. As the interosseous ligament (orange) responds, the joint will open around your fingers.

As the name suggests, your fingertips will form a wedge right at the SIJ. This puts pressure into the spinal erectors, sacral multifides (Figure 13.10), and posterior SI ligaments (all possible sources of SIJ pain). When you are in position, wait here; once the outer layers release, your client's pelvic structure will open and settle around your fingers. This opening is the result of a response in the strong interosseous SI ligaments (Figure 13.8).

Alternatively, use two hands to assess and address both SIJs simultaneously (Figure 13.9). Be aware of your body mechanics, as this position can be more challenging than the one-sided version, though it does allow for precise side-to-side comparisons and a sense of side-to-side balance for your client. Having both sides worked in this

Key Points: Sacroiliac Wedge Technique

Indications include:
- Sacroiliac, low back, or sciatic pain;
- Pain or mobility issues associated with asymmetrical patterns (scoliosis, pelvic asymmetries, leg length differences);
- Preparation for or integration of other work.

Purpose
- Balance any left/right differences in anterior/posterior sacroiliac adaptability (both amplitude and quality of motion);
- Joint hydration and proprioceptive stimulation;
- Calming and quieting (via parasympathetic nervous system responses).

Instructions
- Use SIJ A/P Technique (or other method) to assess differences in left/right SIJ mobility.
- On the less mobile side, use fingertips to press into the joint space. Wait with static pressure for a slight yielding of the tissues over this joint, and a slight widening or softening of the joint itself.

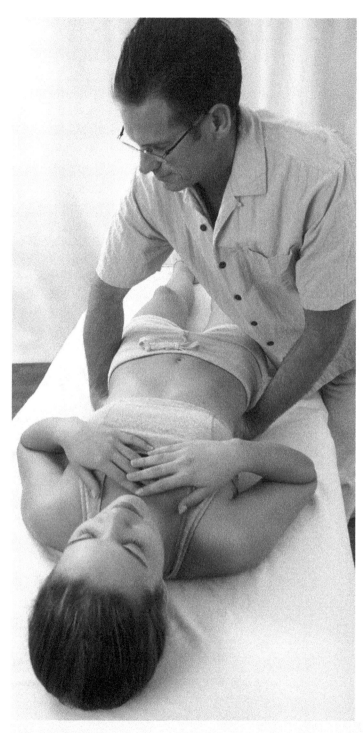

way can be particularly relieving when the SIJs are irritated, perhaps because the bilateral pressure simulates the pressure of sacral multifides contraction (multifides size and the resulting pressure they exert on the sacrum have been observed to be diminished in some cases of lower back pain) (3).

Sacroiliac pain

SIJ pain is frequently the result of an injury, such as a fall or auto accident. One peer-reviewed study showed that about three in five cases of SIJ pain can be traced to a traumatic injury (4). Hormonal changes and pregnancy can bring on SIJ pain, as can arthritis and inflammatory bowel disease. A limp or gait impairment from a knee or ankle issue (for example) can also irritate the SIJ, usually on the opposite side. Asymmetrical forces on the sacrum, such as imbalanced sacrotuberous ligaments (discussed in the previous chapter), iliacus, or rotators, can cause pain and irritation as well.

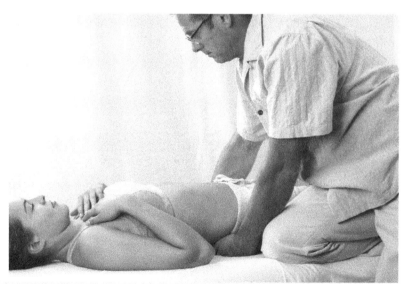

Figures 13.9a/b
The Sacroiliac Wedge Technique, performed bilaterally.

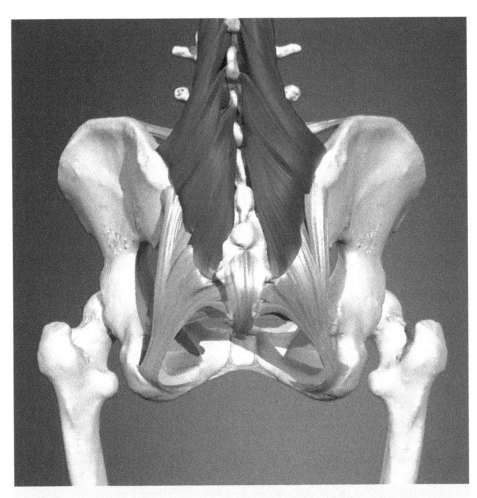

Figure 13.10

The sacral multifides and sacrotuberous ligaments are two of the soft-tissue structures affected by the SIJ techniques.

SIJ pain is often felt by the sufferer to be directly in or superficial to the SIJ; however, because the joints are deep and large, pain related to the SIJs can be hard to localize precisely. SI pain can refer to the hip, groin, buttock, down the leg, or to the low back. Research involving blocking SI sensation with an anesthetic has shown the SIJs to be directly responsible for 15 to 21 percent of generalized low back pain (5). It is likely that the SIJs are indirectly responsible for an even greater percentage of back pain, since the SIJs play such an important role in spinal alignment and mobility.

When there is pain or irritation felt at the SIJ, it is usually unilateral or asymmetrical – that is, worse on one side. As mentioned, the SIJ can be problematic by being either immobile or hypermobile. Pain, sensitivity, and irritation can be felt on either the immobile or hypermobile side, although more severe and ongoing irritation is more commonly felt on the hypermobile side. Even though hands-on work is generally better at loosening than tightening tissues, we can still help hypermobile SIJs in a number of ways. Here are some considerations:

1. If the side that is less mobile is more painful, work to soften that same side, using the techniques discussed here (or others). This usually provides immediate relief, and when incorporated into ongoing work and complementary activities – such as stretching and habit modification – it can provide lasting results.

2. If the side that is more mobile is also more painful, release the opposite (less mobile) side, but do much less work (if any) on the hypermobile, painful joint. Work any soreness in the gluteals and hip muscles on the hypermobile side (since they are likely working to compensate for the lack of ligament stability), but do far less work directly on the hypermobile joint, at least at this stage. Some work here is helpful for joint hydration and propriocep-

tive refinement, but keep it to a minimum on the hypermobile side, until you know more about how your client responds. Ask your client to track any changes in their discomfort in the days after the session. If there is less pain, you are on the right track and probably have relieved the strain on the hypermobile side by spreading the demands of adaptability across both joints, and/or by hydrating irritated joint tissues. Continue working in this way until the irritation subsides.

3. If your hypermobile client reports no change or a worsening of symptoms after working only on the less mobile, less painful side, you may want to discuss the option of working with the hypermobile side directly. Although conventional wisdom says that working directly with inflamed tissues can further aggravate them, I (and others I have compared notes with) have observed marked improvements in SIJ comfort after working directly with a hypermobile, painful SI. Occasionally, there can be a worsening of symptoms in the day or two following the session; more rarely, this can last for several days. Even in these cases, once the immediate aggravation has settled, there is often less pain and aggravation afterwards. This higher-risk, higher-potential-reward approach is appropriate only if both you and your client are informed and comfortable with its implications. Consider factors such as your level of experience and access to supervision and referral practitioners; your client's history, stability, and the potential impact on his or her life and livelihood; and so on. If you or your client is uncomfortable with the prospect that the symptoms may perhaps worsen afterwards, take the cautious route and work directly only on the asymptomatic side, and engage in less, lighter, and indirect work on the symptomatic side.

4. If SI pain persists, referral to a complementary specialist is indicated. Success in dealing with SI pain has been reported by users of physical therapy, Rolfing and structural integration, osteopathy, chiropractic, rehab and functional medicine, and prolotherapy or sclerotherapy (the tightening of loose ligaments by therapeutic scarring), as well as among those who have undergone fluoroscopic injections and fusion surgery. If you have your client's permission, ask their other practitioners about how your work can support and complement their goals. This is a great way to educate yourself and further help your client.

Keep in mind that the worsening of SI symptoms after using the techniques described here is quite rare. When performed properly, these techniques are non-intrusive and have been successfully used by the thousands of practitioners who have trained with us. Whether you use these techniques to begin a session, address SI pain, or to close and integrate, your clients will appreciate your gentle, precise work with their SIJs.

References

[1] Smidt, G.L. et al. Sacroiliac motion for extreme hip positions. A fresh cadaver study. Spine. 22(18). p. 2073–2082. In addition to 4–8mm of PSIS translation, this and other studies cite up to 17° of angular motion at the SIJs.

[2] Damen, L. et al. (2002) The prognostic value of asymmetric laxity of the sacroiliac joints in pregnancy-related pelvic pain. Spine. 27(24). p. 2820–2824.

[3] Krader, D.F. et al. (2000) Correlation Between the MRI Changes in the Lumbar Multifidus Muscles and Leg Pain. Clinical Radiology. 55. p.145–149

[4] Bernard, T.N. et al. (1987) Recognizing specific characteristics of nonspecific low back pain. Clinical Orthopaedics and Related Research. 217. p.266–280.

[5] Lee, D. (2004) The Pelvic Girdle. 3e. Churchill Livingstone.

Picture credits

Figures 13.1, 13.2, 13.7 and 13.10 courtesy Primal Pictures.
Figure 13.3: Image courtesy Thinkstock.
Figures 13.4, 13.5, 13.6 and 13.8, 13.9 courtesy Advanced-Trainings.com.

Study Guide

The Sacroiliac Joints

1   The chapter mentions that the sacrum is one of the body's main locations for _____.

a   nociceptive mechanoreceptors
b   articular hypermobility
c   parasympathetic nerve ganglia
d   sympathetic nerve ganglia

2   The chapter states that the sacroiliac joint articulating planes are oriented _____.

a   coronally
b   sagittally
c   horizontally
d   obliquely

3   What is the stated purpose of the practitioner working from underneath the supine client's sacrum?

a   to rotate the sacrum
b   to lift the sacrum anteriorly
c   to allow the sacrum to drop posteriorly
d   to side bend the sacrum

4   As described in the text, where are the practitioner's fingers lifting in the SI Anterior/Posterior Release Technique?

a   medial to the posterior superior iliac spine on the sacrum
b   lateral to the posterior superior iliac spine on the ilium
c   superior to the posterior superior iliac spine on the ilium
d   inferior to the posterior superior iliac spine on the sacrum

5   The text states that sacroiliac stiffness is highly variable between individuals, but more even side-to-side in:

a   active people
b   asymptomatic people
c   symptomatic people
d   underweight people

For Answer Keys, visit www.Advanced-Trainings.com/v1key/

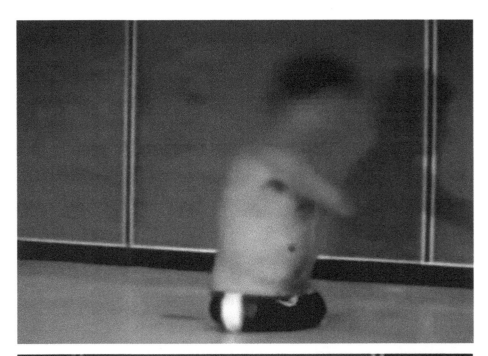

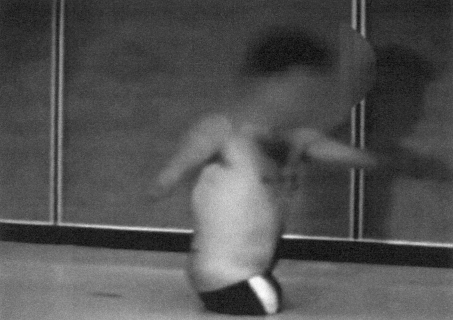

Figures 14.1/14.2

Born without legs, this man walks on his ischial tuberosities by combining rotation of the spine and pelvis, with anterior (14.2) and posterior (14.1) rotation of each innominate bone (made more visible by the white stripe on his clothing).

We walk with our legs. True or false? True. Obviously, as humans, we use our legs to walk. And, false: we use much more than just our legs when walking. In fact, we do not even need legs to walk. Case in point: physicist and spinal researcher Serge Gracovetsky, in his lectures about his influential "Spinal Engine" theory, shows a provocative video of a man born without legs, walking back and forth on his ischial tuberosities instead of his feet. Instead of swinging his legs, the subject rotates his spine and pelvis as he rotates his ilia in opposite directions, alternating one tuberosity in front of the other (Figures 14.1 and 14.2). Gracovetsky's point: whether we have legs or not, we also walk using the inherent mobility of our spine and pelvis.

Gracovetsky's sophisticated theory of spinal energy uptake is not the focus of this chapter, however if you are at all interested in gait, spinal function, or biomechanics, I recommend Web-searching for his talks, or reading his chapter in the textbook, *Dynamic Body: Exploring Form, Expanding Function* edited by Erik Dalton (1). His is one of several influential models that analyze and describe the biomechanics of gait. Most of these theories are intricate and arcane in the extreme; moreover, it does not help that the terminology used varies from author to author, as do basic notions of normal or desirable biomechanics. The nuanced cycle of gait is itself complex: timing, momentum, gravity, weight shift, balance, form- and force-closing of joints, muscle sequencing, proprioceptors, and long chains of osseous and fascial connections all play a part in the seemingly simple miracle of walking.

In this chapter, I will focus on just one key piece of the walking puzzle by describing some straightforward ways to encourage innominate bone mobility.

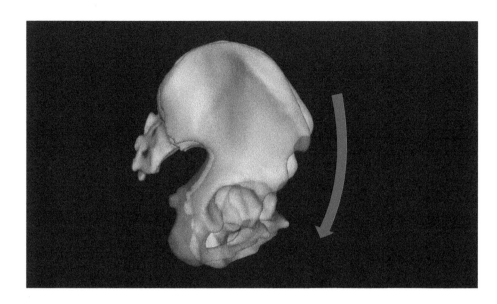

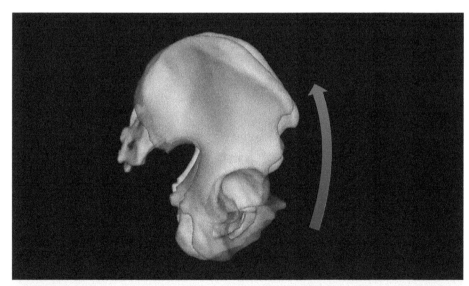

Figures 14.3/14.4

In normal walking, the innominate bone swings in the anterior (14.3) and posterior (14.4) rotation. These movements are also known as anterior and posterior torsion of the innominate. The superimposed innominate images have been rotated 10°; depending on the source, normal motion is thought to be within a range of 2° to 17° of rotation.

Colloquially (but somewhat incorrectly), the term "ilia" is sometimes used as a synonym for the innominate bones (perhaps because the ilia are the most obviously palpated portions of the innominates – for example, when you put your hands on your hips – or because most motion happens at the *sacroiliac* joints). Given its commonality, we will use the convention of calling the innominates "ilia" in this chapter. The techniques described here owe their inspiration to Gracovetsky and others.

Let us begin by making a distinction between two kinds of pelvic movement:

Assess Your Own Ilia Mobility

Here is a simple way to feel innominate bone movement in your own body:

1. Place your hands on your hips, thumbs behind you on your left and right posterior superior iliac spines (PSISs).
2. Slowly, lift one knee. Feel for the movement of each innominate bone (felt as the motion of each PSIS, independent of one another), as opposed to movement of the entire pelvis (felt as both hands moving together).
3. In unrestricted, normal mobility, as you lift your knee, your PSIS on the same (un-weighted) side will drop slightly as the ilium goes into posterior rotation (Figure 14.4).
4. Compare the left and right sides: side-to-side evenness is usually more important than the total amount of movement. Less PSIS drop on one side signals probable restriction of the sacroiliac joint (SIJ) on that same side (although, if there is chronic SIJ pain, it is often on the other, more mobile side). You can adapt this simple assessment for use with clients by comparing left and right PSIS drop as your client lifts each knee in turn. Use the Posterior Rotation Technique to release the less mobile side, and recheck.

1. Movements of the entire pelvic girdle (tucking, shifting, dropping, tilting, rocking, etc.)
2. Intra-segmental movements of the innominate bones and sacrum within the pelvis itself.

Both kinds of pelvic movement occur in walking – the entire pelvis shifts left and right over the standing foot, and so on. Meanwhile, each individual innominate bone also moves within the pelvic girdle, with joint motion occurring at the sacroiliac joints and pubic symphysis (see Assess Your Own Ilia Mobility). This independent motion of the innominates is important because it:

- Acts as a shock absorber in walking, running, and jumping.
- Locks the sacroiliac (SI) joint into a stable position in weight bearing.
- Recycles the energy of gait by loading and releasing the SI ligaments through spring-like recoil.

Limitations in innominate mobility indicate SI joint restriction. When this movement is absent or asymmetrical, local symptoms can include lower back pain, SI joint pain, osteitis pubis (soreness at the pubic symphysis), hip pain, sciatic pain, restricted hip mobility, and more. Loss of movement (hypomobility) of the innominates has global effects as well, and this can be related to knee issues, ankle overpronation, functional scoliosis, and so on. (SI joints can also cause problems when they are hypermobile. For a discussion about working with hypo- and hypermobile SI joints, see the previous chapter, *The Sacroiliac Joints*.)

The amount of innominate movement that should be considered "normal" is a subject of debate, ranging from a low of 2° to a whopping 17° of rotation at the SI (2). As a point of reference, Figures 14.3 and 14.4 show 10° of rotational movement, or about the median value of the

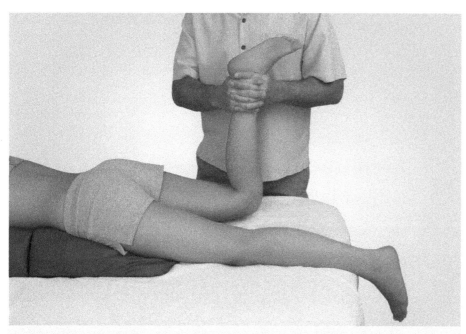

Figure 14.5

The Leg Dangling Technique. Lift just high enough to swing the knee medially and laterally (into hip adduction and abduction). Use this motion to release the hip in preparation for specific work with the innominate and sacroiliac joint.

different published opinions. Other studies suggest that side-to-side evenness is more important than the absolute amount of movement, with pelvic pain more common in individuals with asymmetrical SI stiffness (3).

Leg Dangling Technique

The legs and hips are constantly working whenever we are standing, walking or sitting. Easing the resting tone of the musculature around the hip will help us be more specific and effective when we address the deeper ligamentous SI joint limitations themselves.

With a loose grip around your client's lower leg (Figure 14.5), gently lift the leg just off the table. Do not lift it so high that your client's pelvis tilts and pushes the lumbars into a deeper lordosis; lifting just half an inch (1 cm) off the table is usually enough. Gently swing your client's knee from side to side, feeling for and encouraging release of any muscular tension or holding around the hip. With practice, you will be able to sense and relieve holding and mobility restrictions throughout your client's body with this deceptively simple technique.

Key points: Leg Dangling Technique

Indications include:
- Low back pain, SI joint pain, osteitis pubis, hip pain, sciatic pain, restricted hip mobility, etc.

Purpose
- Assessment and release of any muscular holding of the hip, leg, spine, etc. in preparation for specific innominate mobility techniques.

Instructions
- Suspend one leg slightly off the table, as described in the text. Gently swing (adduct/abduct) the hanging leg to feel for and release any muscular holding in the hip, spine, or elsewhere in the body.

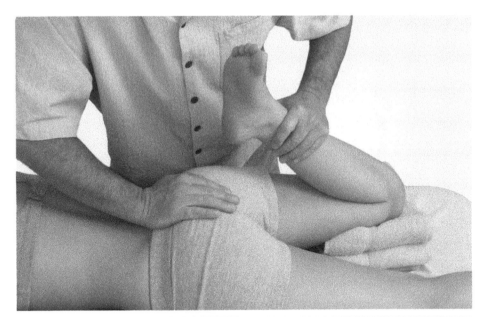

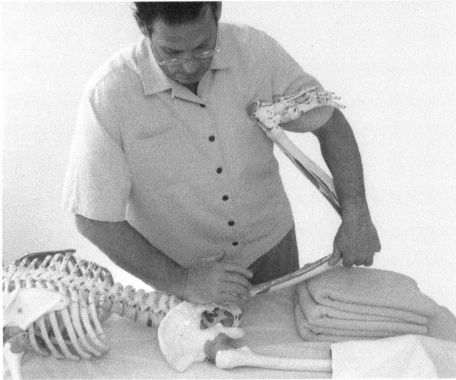

Figures 14.6/14.7

The Anterior Rotation Technique. Use passive hip extension to roll the innominate anteriorly. Use your other hand to stabilize and counter stretch the sacrum caudally or foot-ward. This focuses the motion at the SI joint, and helps free restrictions to anterior innominate rotation. Hip extension can be accomplished with a bolster as in 14.6, or by lifting as in 14.7.

Some clients will find it difficult to relax their leg and simply let it hang. Be patient, and gradually coax the hip into an easier swing. If you find holding or tightness that does not release on its own, you can also address it with more direct techniques such as our "Push Broom" sequence, described in Chapter 10, *Hip Mobility*.

This preparatory assessment has its roots in the approach of bodywork pioneer, Milton Trager MD (1908–1997), and is useful before administering any hip or pelvic work.

Anterior Rotation Technique

See video of the Anterior Rotation Technique at http://advanced-trainings.com/v/pa09.html.

Once you have assessed and addressed the hip's resting tone, you can more easily assess and release any deeper restrictions to anterior innominate rotation (also referred to as anterior rotation of the innominate).

With your client prone, lift one knee to extend the hip, as in Figure 14.7. If your client is larger than you are, you can achieve the same effect by placing the leg on a firm bolster, such as on a stack of sheets (Figure 14.6). In this position of passive hip hyperextension, the pull of the quadriceps rolls the innominate into anterior rotation. Use your other hand on the center of the sacrum to prevent the low back from overextending into an uncomfortable lordosis. Place this second hand on the center of the sacrum and apply firm foot-ward (caudal) pressure (curved arrow, Figure 14.8). This motion of the sacrum (counternutation), together with passive hip extension, focuses the movement into the same-side SI joint.

Wait in this position for the pelvic myofascia and ligaments to adapt and release. Typically, you will take five to eight slow breaths before you feel the subtle drift and yielding that signals this change.

Mobilize both innominates in this way. Alternatively, before doing this technique, you can compare left/right mobility using the Innominate

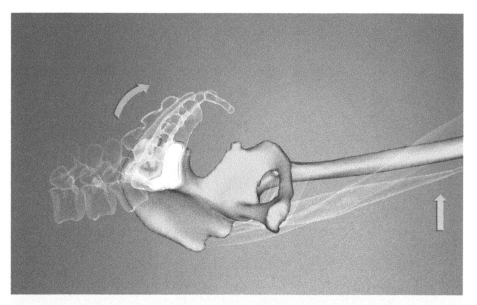

Figure 14.8

The bony movements of the Anterior Rotation Technique. By rolling the innominate anteriorly with the lifted leg (arrows), movement is focused at the SI joint (white).

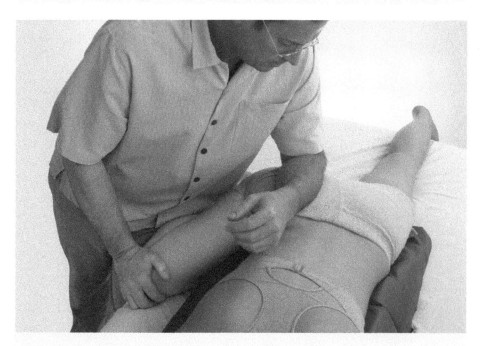

Figure 14.9

The Posterior Rotation Technique, prone variation. Flex the hip as high as comfortable to mobilize posterior rotation of the innominate. Augment the posterior rotation with gentle foot-ward pressure on the PSIS with your forearm. Wait for the slight drift of the hipbone that signals release.

Key points: Anterior Rotation Technique

Indications include:
- Low back pain, SI joint pain, osteitis pubis, hip pain, sciatic pain, restricted hip mobility, etc.

Purpose
- Ensure full range of innominate anterior rotation mobility at the SI joint.

Instructions
1. Assess anterior rotation mobility, comparing left and right sides.
2. Lift or bolster the more restricted-side leg into hip hyperextension, so as to rotate the innominate anteriorly.
3. Apply caudal counter-pressure to the center of the sacrum, taking it into passive counternutation. This focuses the movement at the SI joint.
4. Wait in this position for a myofascial and ligamentous response. Repeat on other side.
5. Finish with Posterior Rotation Technique or similar.

Mobility Assessment (see **"Assess your own ilia mobility"** text box) and focus your work on the more restricted side.

Posterior Rotation Technique

After addressing restrictions to anterior innominate rotation with the previously described technique, integrate and balance your work by making sure the innominates move freely in a complementary direction, into posterior rotation (Figure 14.3).

Bring your client's hip into flexion, either in a prone (Figure 14.9) or supine position. Each position has its advantages; with your client prone, you can use your forearm on the posterior superior iliac spine (PSIS) to gently encourage posterior innominate rotation. This position is easy on the practitioner's body, and is probably preferred when working with clients who are larger than you. In the supine option (not pictured), passively stretch your face-up client's knee towards his or her chest. With one of your hands under the same-side PSIS, apply foot-ward (caudal) traction to that prominence to encourage the desired posterior innominate rotation.

A useful variation for either position is to actively engage the hamstrings and gluteals with a cue such as "Push your leg back down towards straight, against my pressure." Stabilize the leg by continuing to push the knee towards your client's chest, against your client's active hip extension. This isometric muscle-energy approach will use the pull of the muscles that posteriorly rotate the innominate to assist with its mobilization.

Key points: Posterior Rotation Technique

Indications include:
- Low back pain, SI joint pain, osteitis pubis, hip pain, sciatic pain, restricted hip mobility, etc.
- Hypermobile or unstable SI joint.

Purpose
- Ensure full range of innominate posterior rotation mobility at the SI joint.

Instructions
1. Assess posterior rotation mobility, comparing left and right sides.
2. Bring the more-restricted side's hip into flexion. Using your other hand or forearm on the PSIS, encourage posterior rotation with caudal (towards the feet) traction.
3. Alternatively, cue your client to isometrically engage the hamstrings and gluteals with resisted hip extension.
4. Wait in this position for a myofascial and ligamentous response. Repeat on other side.

Movement
- Optionally, use active isometric (resisted) hip extension to further pull the innominate into posterior rotation. "Push your leg back down towards straight, against my pressure."

As in the anterior rotation technique, wait for several breaths with either the passive or active variation, until you feel a slight drifting or yielding of the innominate in the desired posterior direction; then, recheck for side-to-side balance.

Both the prone and supine positions use the pull of the hamstrings in hip flexion to roll the innominate farther into posterior rotation. If this important motion is restricted, the SI joint may not reach the close-packed position it needs for fully stable weight bearing. For this reason, it is usually preferable to do this technique after freeing up anterior rotation, so as to leave clients with the stable, solid feeling that full posterior rotation can bring.

Finish your work by linking the two sides of the body in your client's awareness. For example, use the bilateral SI Wedge Technique (see Chapter 13, *The Sacroiliac Joints*) to balance the left and right sides of the sacrum. Additionally, it's a good idea to finish with some kind of neck work, since addressing the other end of the spine helps complement the focused pelvic work just performed.

References

[1] Dalton, E. et al. (2011) *Dynamic Body: Exploring Form, Expanding Function.* Freedom From Pain Institute; 1st edition.

[2] Buyruk, H.M. (1995) Measurements of sacroiliac joint stiffness with colour Doppler imaging: A study on healthy subjects. *Eur. J. Radiol.* 21. p. 117–122.

[3] Damen, L. et al. (2002) The prognostic value of asymmetric laxity of the sacroiliac joints in pregnancy-related pelvic pain. *Spine.* (Phila Pa 1976). Dec 15; 27(24). p. 2820–2824.

Picture credits

Figures 14.1 and 14.2 courtesy Dr. Serge Gracovetsky. Used with permission.
Figures 14.3, 14.4 and 14.8 courtesy Primal Pictures. Used with permission.
Figures 14.5, 14.6, 14.7 and 14.9 courtesy Advanced-Trainings.com.

Study Guide

The Ilia

1　According to the text, what do innominate mobility limitations indicate?

　a　muscle imbalances
　b　ligamentous damage
　c　gait problems
　d　sacroiliac joint restrictions

2　What does the text state that the practitioner is feeling for with the Leg Dangling Technique?

　a　sacroiliac ligamentous release
　b　muscular tonus release
　c　posterior ilia rotation release
　d　anterior ilia rotation release

3　According to the text, what hip position does the practitioner use in the Anterior Rotation Technique?

　a　extension
　b　flexion
　c　abduction
　d　external rotation

4　According to the text, when assessing ilia mobility by lifting one knee, the same-side PSIS will move in which way if ilia mobility is unrestricted?

　a　move laterally
　b　move up
　c　not move at all
　d　move down

5　In what direction is the forearm pressure in the Posterior Rotation Technique?

　a　foot-ward on the sacrum
　b　head-ward on the sacrum
　c　foot-ward on the PSIS
　d　head-ward on the PSIS

For Answer Keys, visit www.Advanced-Trainings.com/v1key/

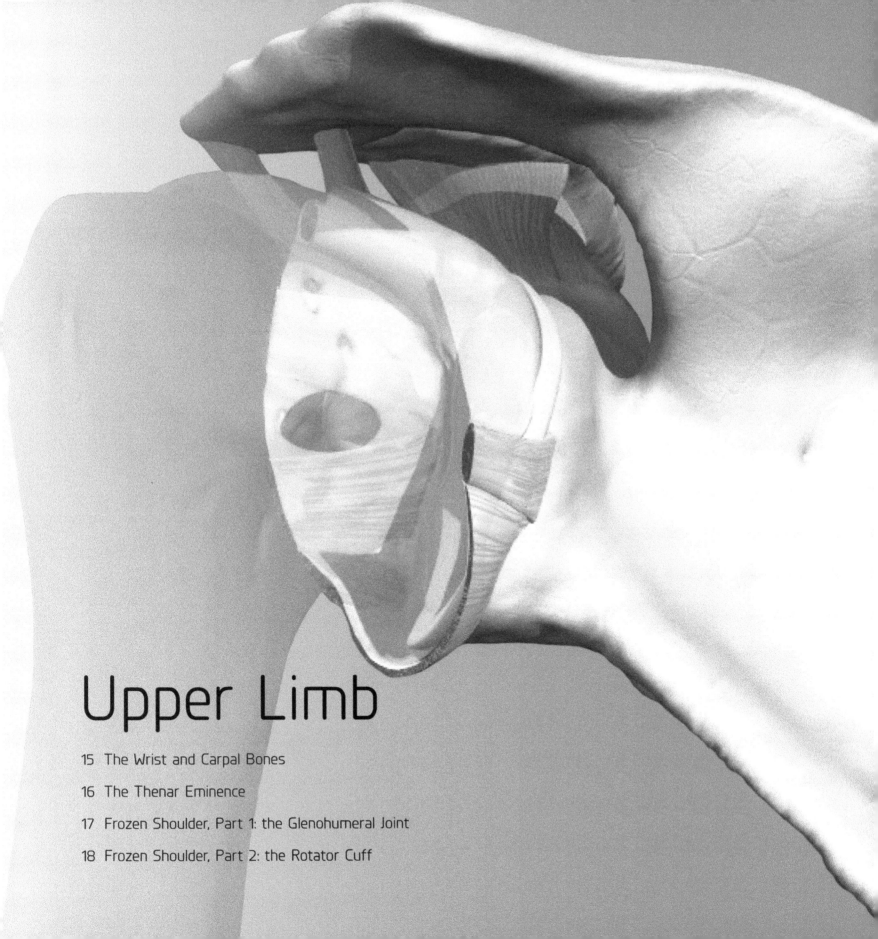

Upper Limb

The Wrist and Carpal Bones

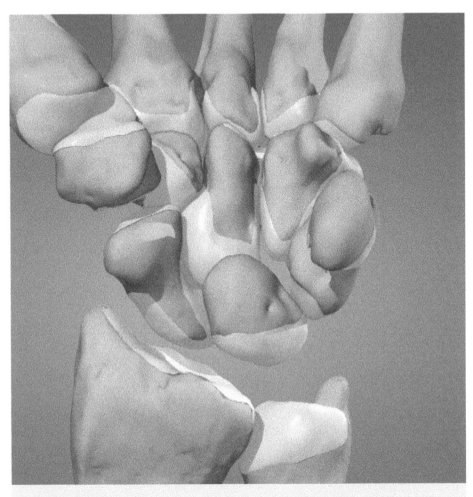

Figure 15.1a

The structure of the wrist balances movement and stability, combining slippery articular cartilage (white areas), synovial joints, and a strong system of interlocking ligaments between the carpal bones (15.1b). Loss of movement between the carpal bones can be associated with the symptoms of carpal tunnel syndrome, arthritis, wrist pain, and diminished hand function.

Wrists are marvelous structures. They mediate the relationship between our stable larger-boned arms and the highly mobile, sensitive dexterity of our small-boned hands. Additionally, key structures pass through the wrists on their way from the arms to the hands: tendons, nerves, and vessels. In this chapter, I will describe two effective techniques for working with the wrist.

The carpus is the bony structure formed by the two rows of the small carpal bones. Wherever these bones meet each other, they have slippery hyaline cartilage and fluid-filled synovial joints between them. They are also secured by a complex system of strong interlocking ligaments (Figure 15.1b). In other words, the carpus bones are built to provide both mobility and stability. By combining these two qualities, the integrated structure of the carpus provides a stable yet adaptable base for the varied movements of the hand, fingers, and thumb.

Problems can occur when either mobility is lost (hypo-mobility) or when stability is lost (hyper-mobility). Hypo-mobility issues can arise from several causes, including past injuries that have self-splinted as they healed; surgeries; arthritic conditions; and/or soft-tissue adaptations to heavy or repetitive work. Generally speaking, hyper-mobility issues are usually the result of injury or congenital conditions. Typically, manual therapy practitioners will see more clients who present with issues related to a lack of mobility than clients who present with too much mobility, and so the techniques described here will focus on providing more mobility. However, even clients with hyper-mobile patterns will usually have local areas of hypo-mobility. With these clients, you can help restore the overall balance of the wrist by applying these techniques to the articulations where there is less motion.

Referral to an orthopedist, physical therapist, occupational therapist, or other medical professional who specializes in hand issues is, of course, indicated for serious recent or unresolved injuries, or when your client has ongoing symptoms that you think might be related to overly mobile wrist joints.

Lost carpal mobility can play a role in the numbness and pain of carpal tunnel compression symptoms. Together with the bowstring-like flexor retinaculum, the bowed arch of the carpus forms the carpal tunnel – the space through which the tendons, vessels, and nerves of the hand pass.

Structurally, it is all too easy for the contents of this tunnel to become crowded and irritated, especially in wrist extension. Although there are many factors that can contribute to carpal tunnel narrowing, in my practice, I have unscientifically observed that a less mobile capitate bone (Figure 15.4) is often found in people with pain and carpal tunnel symptoms. It follows to reason that if the capitate is unable to move dorsally with wrist extension, the carpal tunnel flattens, and neurovascular compression symptoms of pain, weakness, and numbness can be more likely to occur, especially in the median nerve distribution area of the thumb pad and the ends of fingers two to three (1).

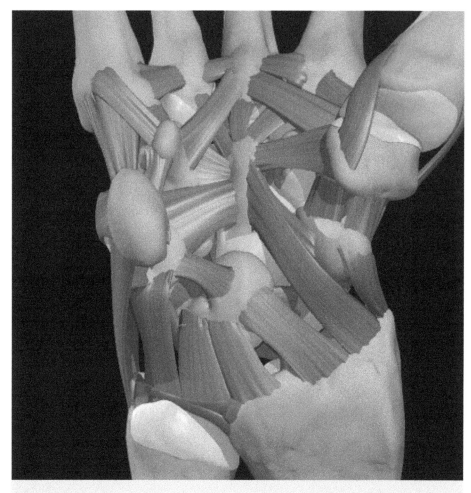

Figure 15.1b

The structure of the wrist balances movement and stability, combining slippery articular cartilage (white areas), synovial joints, and a strong system of interlocking ligaments between the carpal bones (15.1b). Loss of movement between the carpal bones can be associated with the symptoms of carpal tunnel syndrome, arthritis, wrist pain, and diminished hand function.

See video of the Carpal Mobility Technique at http://advanced-trainings.com/v/aa04.html.

Carpal Mobility Technique

Our first step will be to assess the mobility of the carpal bones. With a firm grip on the carpus, as shown in Figure 15.2, move individual carpal bones against one another in an anterior/posterior (A/P) direction (in the hand, this is referred to as dorsal/volar motion). Firmly but gently "scrub" all the carpal bones against one another, much like you would if you were scrubbing a stain in a piece of clothing. Be thorough, moving each of the carpal articulations in turn.

In this technique, feel specifically for the bones. Instead of working only with soft tissue, we are feeling for the mobility of the carpal bones themselves. There is no kneading, petrissage, traction, or wrist stretching in this technique – focus instead on encouraging carpal movement in the A/P dimension. Be slow, full, and sensitive; but your touch can be quite firm (as long as it is comfortable for your client and he or she is not recovering from an injury or instability issue). Lean into it, and wait for a release at the end-range in each direction. Be sure to keep your own hands as soft and adaptable as possible.

When working with people who use their hands for heavy or repetitive work, or with those with wrist pain, you will often find one or two areas that are particularly immobile, as if two or three of the carpal bones had fixed themselves into a non-moving "coalition." Often, these coalitions involve the central carpals (particularly the trapezoid, scaphoid, and/or the capitate). As mentioned, the capitate is in a position to be particularly troublesome to the carpal tunnel, so be sure it is as mobile as possible, especially in a posterior or dorsal direction.

For a variation of this technique, you can passively flex, extend, and side-bend your client's wrist as you monitor A/P carpal motion. Since the carpal tunnel tends to narrow with wrist extension, checking carpal mobility in an extended position can reveal restrictions that are easy to miss in a neutral wrist position.

Incidentally, the proximal row of carpal bones usually has more inter-carpal movement than the distal row to allow for the adaptability needed for movement between the hand and arm bones. The comparatively greater stability of the distal row plays a role in maintaining the carpal tunnel's space, but as a result, the distal row is more prone to being fixed and hypo-mobile.

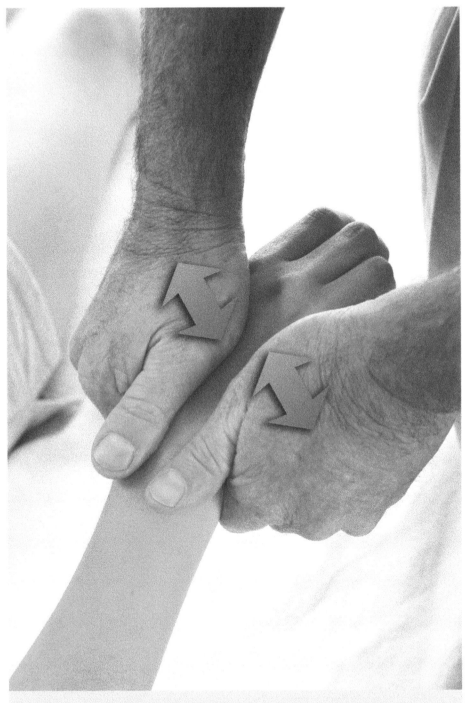

Figure 15.2

In the Carpal Mobility Technique, use a firm "scrubbing" movement to check and release anterior/posterior (volar/dorsal) movement of each carpal articulation.

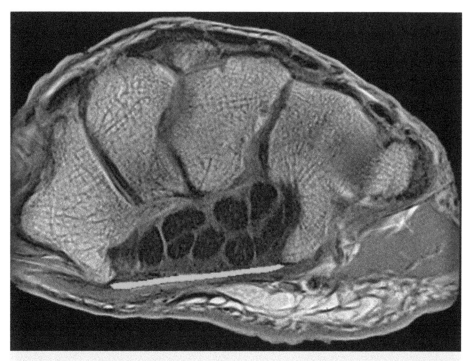

Figure 15.3

A magnetic resonance image (MRI) cross-section of the distal carpal bones, with the flexor retinaculum in green. Note the tightly packed arrangement of the tendons, nerves, and vessels squeezing through the carpal tunnel.

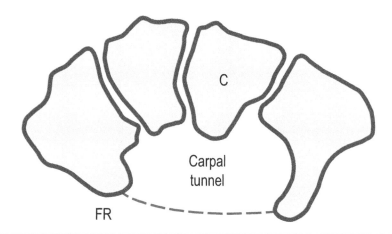

Figure 15.4

The distal row of the carpus and the carpal tunnel, in cross-section. The flexor retinaculum, on the palm side, is labeled FR. The capitates bone (C) is prone to being fixed anteriorly (or volar, towards the palm), thus contributing to carpal tunnel narrowing.

Once you have thoroughly checked and released A/P carpal mobility, you can use the next technique to make sure that the carpal tunnel itself is as open as possible.

Key points: Carpal Mobility Technique

Indications include:
- Wrist or hand immobility or pain, including carpal tunnel and neurovascular compression symptoms.

Purpose
- Differentiate and balance the anterior/posterior mobility of the carpal and metacarpal bones.

Instructions
1. Assess anterior/posterior mobility of each carpal and metacarpal bone in relation to its neighbors.
2. Hold any motion-restricted bones at the end-range of the more-restricted direction. Wait for a softening response. Recheck.

Movements
- Passively flex, extend, and sidebend client's wrist; recheck and release A/P carpal mobility in each position.

Transverse Arch Technique

The Transverse Arch Technique is an effective way to open up more space in a crowded carpal tunnel, and to give your clients a sense of how to maintain this space as they go about their daily activities.

We will return to the image of the carpal bones forming a bow, with the flexor retinaculum serving as the bow's string (Figure 15.4). Since many wrist problems come from the bow being too flat (thus crowding its contents), we want to avoid lengthening or stretching the bowstring, which would further flatten the transverse arch. For this reason, it is often best to avoid direct work right on the flexor retinaculum in clients with neurovascular compression symptoms.

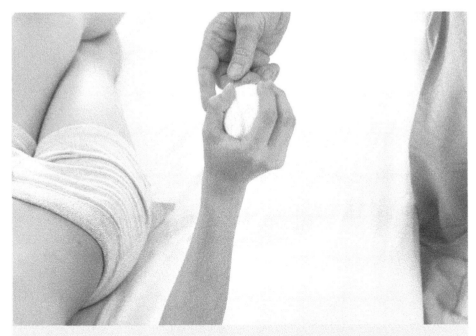

Figure 15.5

The Transverse Arch Technique uses a ball to maintain the concave shape of your client's hand. Invite your client to experiment with letting the whole hand contact the ball by softening rather than squeezing.

Instead, look for ways to widen or open up the "top" (the dorsum) of the arch by encouraging more space in the dorsal aspect of the inter-carpal joints.

Key points: Transverse Arch Technique

Indications include:
- Wrist or hand immobility or pain, including carpal tunnel and neurovascular compression symptoms, particularly when exacerbated by wrist extension.

Purpose
- Ensure transverse arch adaptability and depth of carpal tunnel.
- Refine client's proprioceptive sense of carpal tunnel depth, especially in wrist extension.

Instructions
1. Educate client's proprioceptive sense using a ball, as described in text.
2. Gently work the ligaments at the dorsal intercarpal joints to increase arch depth and enhance proprioception.
3. Assess and release any restrictions to appropriate carpal/radius mobility in full wrist extension, as well as full radial and ulnar deviation.

Movements
- Passively flex, extend, and sidebend client's wrist; recheck and release dorsal intercarpal and carpal/radial mobility in each position.

Client education

This technique has two stages: an educational step that you will guide your client through, and a hands-on manipulation technique.

Give your client a ball that she can wrap her hand around – a tennis ball is a good size for most adults. Ask her to see how much of her hand she can bring into contact with the ball (Figure 15.5). At this point, most people will squeeze the ball tighter, which does indeed bring

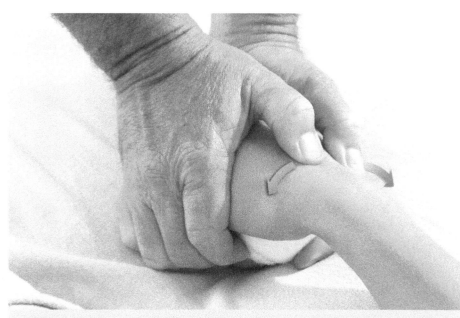

Figure 15.6

Encourage lateral opening of the dorsal intercarpal joints. Work in the direction of the arrows, feeling for a change in bony mobility, rather than simply sliding over the surface.

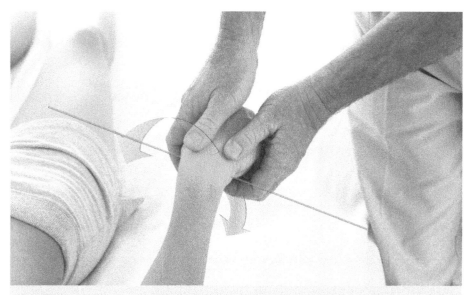

Figure 15.7

With the ball still in your client's hand, add passive wrist movement to the Transverse Arch Technique. This will help you make sure that the back of the wrist can stay wide in various positions. Check wrist flexion/extension (pictured), side-to-side deviation, and their combinations.

more of the hand in contact with the ball, but it also tightens the hand and crowds the carpal tunnel. We are looking for a deep transverse arch without undue tightness or closing, so ask your client to see if, instead of squeezing, she can relax her hand in order to bring more of its surface in contact with the ball. Have her take her time with this; if you help your client stay with it, she will begin to notice more and more subtlety and possibility as she settles in. It can be helpful to draw your client's attention to the rest of her body's response to this exercise – when the hand relaxes around the ball, shoulders typically drop, the breath deepens, the jaw unclenches, and so on. Try it yourself: how much of your hand can you bring in contact with a tennis ball without squeezing or tightening?

This is a useful exercise for anyone, but if your client is dealing with carpal tunnel symptoms, you can explain that the practice of allowing her hand to stay rounded and relaxed in this way can help mitigate the wrist crowding that gives rise to the pain, weakness, and numbness of her carpal tunnel symptoms (2).

Hands-on Manipulation

In the hands-on stage of this technique, ask your client to hold the ball in the relaxed way described above. Then, use your thumbs or fingers to mold her hand around the shape of the ball – you will see or feel where her hand has a harder time relaxing into a concave transverse arch. In particular, feel for a slight opening or softening between the carpal bones on the posterior or dorsal side of the wrist. Gently work the ligaments at the intercarpal joints to bring mobility and enhance proprioception to these important spaces (Figure 15.6).

As in the Carpal "Scrubbing" technique, you can do a variation of the Transverse Arch technique by adding passive wrist motion (Figure 15.7).

While doing the techniques as described, gently take your client's wrist into extension, feeling for the ability of the back of the wrist to stay wide; that is, feel for lateral release at the deep dorsal intercarpal joints. To encourage a full transverse arch, allow the middle carpals to move dorsally (posterior) on the radius, but encourage the outer edges of the carpus to wrap anteriorly around the ball. Feel for flexion and extension at the midcarpal joint, which is the formed by the articulation of the proximal and distal rows of the carpal bones. The side-to-side "royal wave" of radial and ulnar deviation occurs mainly at the radiocarpal joint, and during these movements, you can feel a healthy carpus moving as an integrated but flexible unit. Check each of these motions and their combinations, feeling for and releasing any soft tissue restrictions that seem to be inhibiting the desired concave shape of the hand.

Walking our talk

Just like the cobbler's shoeless children, as hands-on manual therapists, we can tend to neglect our own hand and wrist mobility. Since we use our hands so much in our work, we are particularly prone to losing adaptability in our own carpal joints.

Receiving the kind of work described here is great preventative maintenance, and it can even increase the quality of your work. Although lost mobility may or may not cause overt symptoms, it will cause your touch to feel harder, more rigid, and less comfortable to your clients. It can also take a toll on your sensitivity and dexterity. Your work will be better with adaptable carpal joints.

We have focused our discussion on bones and bony relationships. There are, of course, many factors in wrist issues and carpal tunnel syndrome, but together, the two techniques we have described here can help you get even better results with hand, wrist, and carpal tunnel issues. Do not put off receiving them yourself.

References

[1] There are many good sources for more information about carpal tunnel issues, diagnostic tests, and compression symptoms. Two classics are:
- Cailliet, R. (1996) *Soft Tissue Pain and Disability 3rd edition*. Philadelphia: F.A. Davis, p. 310–329.
- Cailliet, R. (1994) *Hand Pain and Impairment 4th edition*. Philadelphia: F.A. Davis, p. 176–186.

[2] Thanks to Rolfers Judith Aston and Siana Goodwin for their ideas and influences seen in the "ball" technique.

Picture credits

Figures 15.1 and 15.3 courtesy Primal Pictures. Used with permission.
Figure 15.4 courtesy Advanced-Trainings.com (after Kapandji)
Figures 15.2, 15.5, 15.6 and 15.7 courtesy Advanced-Trainings.com

Study Guide

The Wrist and Carpal Bones

1   Which of the below is listed as a possible contributing factor for wrist hypermobility?

a   arthritic conditions
b   surgery
c   soft tissue adaptations
d   injury

2   According to the text, what type of tissue is the practitioner feeling for in the Carpal Mobility Technique?

a   ligament
b   muscle
c   periosteum
d   bone

3   Which bone does the author single out as a contributor to carpal tunnel narrowing?

a   capitate
b   trapezoid
c   scaphoid
d   pisiform

4   In which wrist position is the carpal tunnel most likely, according to the text, to become crowded?

a   flexion
b   side bending
c   extension
d   rotation

5   In the client education stage of the Transverse Arch Technique, what is the function of the ball?

a   massage the client's hand
b   deepen the transverse arch
c   strengthen the wrist muscles
d   differentiate the wrist fascia

For Answer Keys, visit www.Advanced-Trainings.com/v1key/

The Thenar Eminence

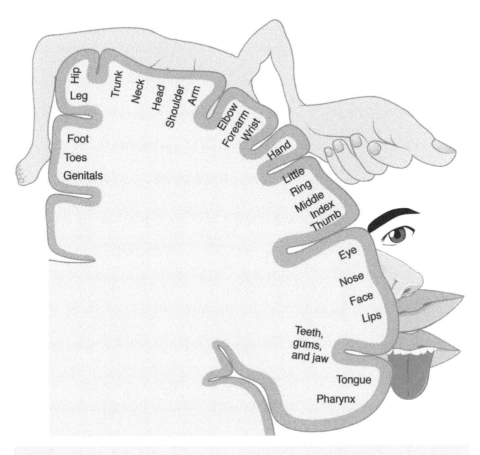

Figure 16.1
The thumb figures large in the brain – an outsized proportion of the sensory homunculus (depicted here) is dedicated to processing thumb sensations. This makes the thumb very sensitive, dexterous, and hard to ignore when painful.

Thank goodness for the thumb. Its unique opposability allows us to grasp, hold, squeeze, and manipulate. Its enormous strength gives power to our grip and its unmatched sensitivity (matched by a colossal portion of the brain dedicated to its sensations) helps us feel the most minute differences in texture, size, or pressure (Figure 16.1).

Thumbs are so good at so many things, that they are very commonly overused, causing tissue and joint irritation, pain, and eventual damage. For example, the increasing use of small-device keyboards means that thumbs are more active than ever in awkward, repetitive movement patterns needed to type out texts, emails, and tweets (Figure 16.2). Some practitioners in our field have taken this as a business opportunity, catering to their business clientele with "Android Thumb," "iPhone Thumb," and "gamer's thumb" manual therapy hand treatments designed to ease the strain and pain of excessive thumb keyboarding.

However, manual therapists themselves are, of course, vulnerable to thumb over-reliance – in our Advanced Myofascial Techniques seminars, we see practitioners in every workshop who are dealing with the effects of thumb overuse, and sometimes these cases are severe (see *A few rules of thumb below* for a few ways to avoid excessive thumb use).

The structure of the thumb lends it special qualities, and predisposes it to unique vulnerabilities. The thumb's joints are the most mobile of all the digits, allowing the thumb its distinctive opposability and adaptability. As with the fingers, articular ligaments provide some stability, but because of its highly mobile joints, the thumb gets most of its stability from coordinated, active muscular tension. The muscles of the thumb are arrayed

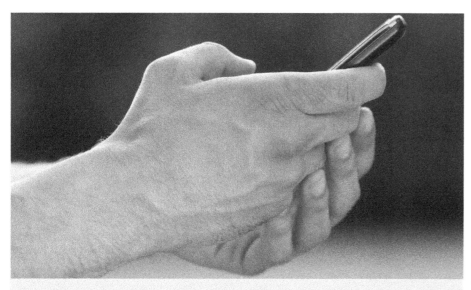

Figure 16.2

"Android Thumb" is another name for the increasingly common thumb/thenar-eminence pain and irritation resulting from excessive use of small keyboards and controls.

in all directions around it, like guy-wires around a pole or mast (Figure 16.3). Moreover, these muscles stay busy; given that so much of the thumb's stability comes from the tension of these muscles, most thumb muscles are active during most thumb movements (1). It is no wonder our thumbs get tired.

A Few Rules of Thumb

There are a few principles for sustainable thumb use:

- The best way to use your thumbs is usually to use something else instead. The most sustainable thumb alternatives are bony projections such as your forearm, soft fist (Figure 16.9), or knuckle. With practice and creative positioning, any of these tools can be as sensitive and as specific as your thumb.
- Avoid hyperextension (Figure 16.8) at any of your thumb joints. Hyperextension may feel stable, but this stability relies on stretching your articular ligaments and joint capsules to their maximum length, which will cause them to slacken over time. This leads to less stability and eventual pain.
- A neutral joint position is good; even better is to keep a small amount of flexion at each thumb joint. Engaging the powerful flexor muscles of your palm will support your thumb joints and ligaments. If this positioning is not familiar, you may need to practice it gradually as you develop the necessary flexor strength. You do not actually need much strength, but you do need a little, and if you are not accustomed to working with slightly flexed thumb joints, the muscles involved may be quite weak at first.
- Pain or discomfort is a sign that something is wrong. If your thumb or hand hurts when doing a technique, do it in a different way. This sounds obvious, but many of us forget about our own comfort when we are focused on that of our clients.
- Some practitioners have found hand-held tools or thumb splints useful. I have not, but you might.

When using a hand-held tool, be sure that you are acutely attuned to your client's verbal and non-verbal signals, since you have less direct tactile feedback with a tool.

- Save your thumbs for the few places where they excel and are truly irreplaceable. After several thumb injuries unrelated to bodywork, and after 30 years of manual therapy practice, I still use my thumbs quite comfortably (knock on wood) in a few areas. In addition to the Thenar Eminence Technique, I use my thumbs for working the 1) iliolumbar ligaments; 2) knee (meniscal ligaments, infrapatellar fat pad, and patellar tendon); and 3) sacrotuberous ligaments (see Chapter 12, The Sacrotuberous Ligaments) – but hardly anywhere else. That is the way that I have found to make them last.

The origins of the word "thumb" go back to the Old English word *thūma*, from the Indo-European word *tum* or "swelling" (which also gave us "tumor" and "thigh"). The swelling in the thumb's case is thought to be its round shape, or the thumb's rounded thenar eminence (the muscular portion of the palm at the base of the thumb). It is here that I will focus our discussion, as the thenar eminence often takes the brunt of thumb overuse and repetitive strain. There are at least two reasons for this:

1. Since the thenar eminence contains the primary muscles involved in finger-to-thumb gripping, activities or occupations that involve repeated or prolonged use of small instruments or fine tools (dentistry, electronic manufacturing, handwriting, and so on) can be associated with thenar eminence overdevelopment, fatigue, and pain.
2. Since its three constituent muscles (abductor pollicis brevis, flexor pollicis brevis, and opponens pollicis) are some of the thumb's bulkiest, the thenar eminence also provides the lion's share of palm-to-thumb grip

strength (for example, when using large tools such as hammers, shovels, or in manual therapy techniques involving squeezing or kneading).

The carpal tunnel connection

Overuse of the thenar eminence is also intimately connected to neurovascular compression and the symptoms of carpal tunnel syndrome (such as hand, palm, or wrist pain, numbness, and tingling). Because all three of its muscles have direct connective tissue continuity with the carpal tunnel's flexor retinaculum (Figure 16.4), repeated or heavy use of the thenar muscles can contribute to tension, strain, or shortness of this carpal ligament, which may narrow the carpal tunnel space and compress its contents.

This thenar eminence/carpal tunnel connection works in both directions – the thenar muscles can contribute to tunnel compression, and tunnel compression can cause thenar pain. While most palm muscles are innervated by the ulnar nerve (which does not pass through the carpal tunnel), the muscles of the thenar eminence are typically innervated by the median nerve (which does pass through the carpal tunnel (Figure 16.4)). Compression of this median nerve is most often responsible for the pain of carpal tunnel syndrome (Chapter 15, *The Wrist and Carpal Bones*). In fact, thenar eminence pain is one of the most common effects of median nerve compression, and atrophy of these muscles (particularly of the flexor pollicis brevis; Figure 16.6) is a possible long-term result of unresolved carpal tunnel neurovascular compression. Direct myofascial manipulation of the thenar eminence has been anecdotally observed to lessen carpal tunnel compression symptoms (1) but if you notice atrophy accompanied by pain here, referral to a rehabilitative specialist is probably indicated. It is also important to remember that median nerve compression symptoms can be related to compression anywhere along the median nerve's length, from the cervical nerve roots, distally through the

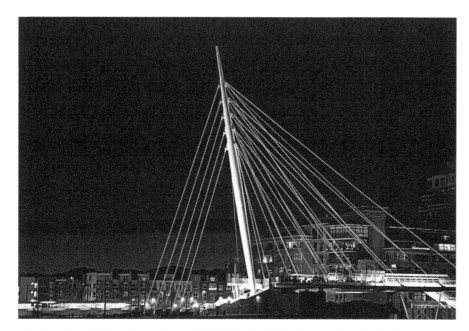

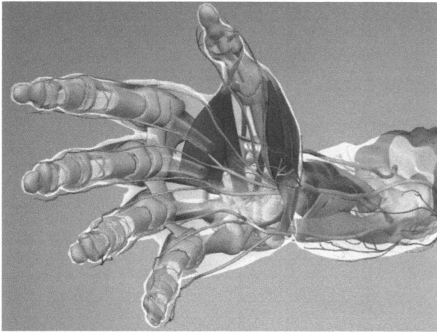

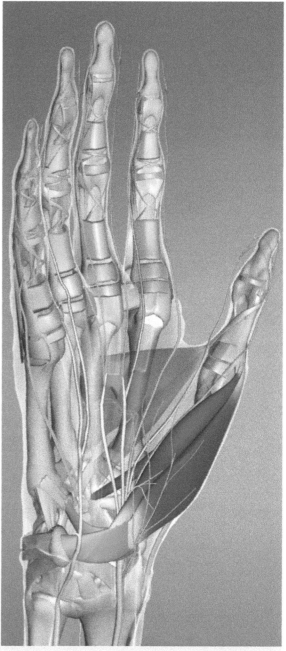

Figures 16.3/16.4/16.5

The thumb's strength and stability comes from the guy-wire-like arrangement of the thenar eminence muscles (16.4 and 16.5), together with the deeper adductor pollicis brevis (semitransparent in 16.4). Also in 16.5, note the continuity of the thenar eminence muscles with the carpal tunnel's flexor retinaculum (orange). The median (right) and ulnar (left) nerves (yellow) are also pictured.

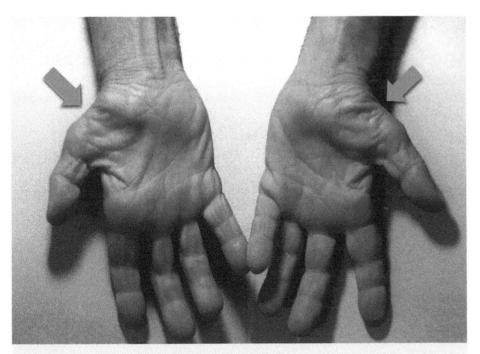

Figure 16.6
Thenar eminence/flexor pollicis brevis atrophy (arrows) as a result of untreated median nerve compression.

brachial plexus, or in the arm, elbow, or forearm – not just in the wrist or hand.

Thenar Eminence Technique

While it is particularly important to keep a global perspective with carpal tunnel symptoms, these symptoms are not the only reason why we should work the thenar eminence. Almost anyone who uses his or her hands will truly appreciate focused local work with the structures of the thumb's base.

See video of the Thenar Eminence Technique at http:// advanced-trainings. com/v/aa05.html.

The first variation of the Thenar Eminence Technique (Figure 16.7) uses the practitioner's thumbs to feel into and release the various layers of the palm. Be sure to use your own thumbs in a way that is comfortable and sustainable. In particular, avoid any hyperextension by maintaining a bit of flexion in each of your thumb joints.

Work from the center of the palm outwards, starting superficially with the palmar fascia and then working deeper, layer-by-layer, until you are deep within the thenar eminence. Although there is some sliding involved, I suggest not using oil or lotion, as the friction will actually provide therapeutic stretching to the palmar and muscular fascias – it should not be uncomfortable if you work slowly enough. As always, be sure your pressure is not too painful for your client. If he or she is gripping or contracting elsewhere in the body as a result of your pressure or speed, you are working against yourself. Slow down and let the layers melt away. Think about how much of the brain's sensory cortex this little area occupies (Figure 16.1) – why rush it?

Once you have engaged a fascial layer, ask for slow, active client movement; some examples include, "Let your hand open, and close," or "Open your thumb." This will slide and differentiate the tissue layers under your pressure, and give clients control over the technique's intensity. Work thoroughly, all through the thenar eminence fascia and the palmar side of the thumb itself, from the superficial to deeper layers, in each place.

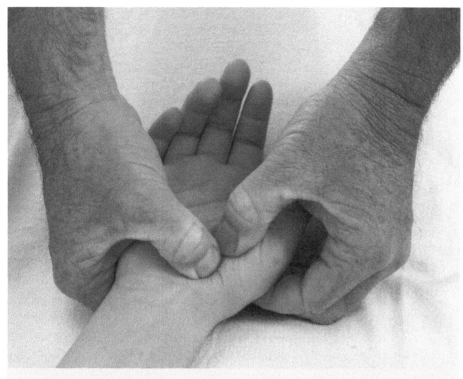

Figure 16.7

The Thenar Eminence Technique. Slowly and patiently work into the structures of the thenar eminence. Add active client thumb and finger movements in order to separate tissue layers. Keep a small amount of flexion in each joint of your own thumbs.

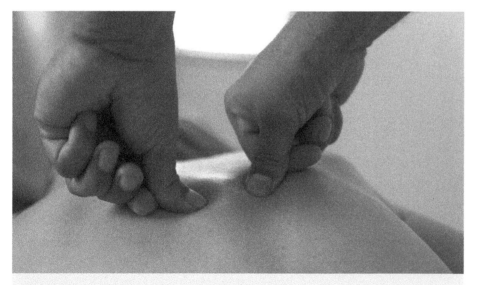

Figure 16.8

Hyperextension of any of the thumb's joints can strain articular ligaments, eventually reducing joint stability.

The second variation of the Thenar Eminence Technique (Figure 16.9) is similar, but it uses the knuckles of the practitioner's soft fist rather than the thumbs. Note that a soft fist is open, not closed. A soft fist is more sensitive and adaptable than a hard, closed fist. In a soft fist, hand stability is achieved by aligning the arm, carpal, and metacarpal bones, rather than by gripping the muscles. This means that the wrist must be in a neutral or very slightly flexed position; however, like the thumb joints, the wrist is never extended.

With your non-working hand, cradle your client's hand from below (Figure 16.9). This will provide you with extra sensitivity and control, as you can tune the position of your client's hand to allow the soft fist to engage just the right layer. The release is performed with your soft fist's MPJ joints (the proximal metacarpal phalangeal joints at the base of the fingers). Use these knuckles to feel into the hand's layers, as in the first variation. With the broader tool of the fist, you can anchor larger sheets of palmar fascia – again asking your client to actively open his or her hand once you have anchored into the desired layer. As in the first variation, be patient and thorough, and include this technique within a whole-limb, whole-body, and whole-person perspective.

If symptoms continue to be troublesome, a shift in your approach or in the client's habits is probably indicated. Given that the thumbs are so active, you may find that clients with occupations or activities that demand a lot from their thumbs may need this kind of work on a regular basis in a maintenance and prevention capacity.

Of course, the soft-fist version of the Thenar Eminence Technique is especially suited to bodyworker self-care. At the end of your day just lay your own hand down on the table and lean into your thenar eminence with the knuckles of your soft fist (or your elbow). Slowly open and close your "client" hand, releasing any thumb tension and fatigue. This would be a great time to say a silent "thank you" for the wonder of thumbs – thank goodness we have them.

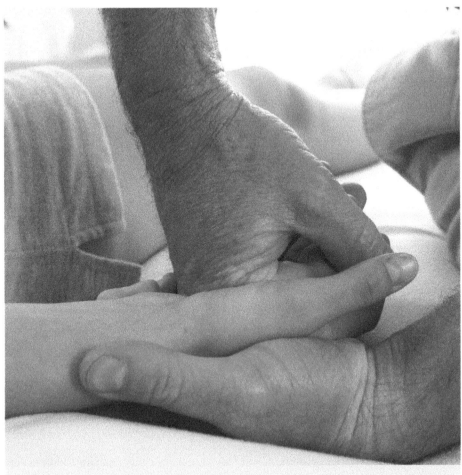

Figure 16.9

Another variation of the Thenar Eminence Technique using the knuckles of a soft fist. Ask your client to slowly open and close her hand to augment the release.

Key points: Thenar Eminence Technique

Indications include:

- Thumb, hand, or wrist pain, including carpal tunnel and neurovascular compression symptoms.
- Pain, weakness, and contracture of overuse conditions such as "Blackberry Thumb," "gamer's thumb," or De Quervain syndrome.

Purpose

- Differentiate and restore elasticity in the fasciae, tendons, and musculature of the thenar eminence and palm.

Instructions

- Use thumbs (carefully) or the knuckles of a soft fist to anchor the tissues of the thenar eminence, starting superficially, then working deeper. Employ active thumb extension and adduction to move the tissues under the practitioner's static touch.

Movements

- Active thumb extension, abduction, and adduction. "Let your hand open, and close," or "Open your thumb, as if you're hitchhiking."

References

[1] Austin, N.M. (2005). Chapter 9: The Wrist and Hand Complex. In Levangie, Pamela K.; Norkin, Cynthia C. Joint Structure and Function: A Comprehensive Analysis (4th ed.). Philadelphia: F. A. Davis Company.

[2] Goodwin, S. (2003) Carpal Tunnel Syndrome and Repetitive Stress Injuries. Massage & Bodywork, December/January.

Picture credits

Figure 16.1 "1421 Sensory Homunculus" by OpenStax College - Anatomy & Physiology, Connexions. Licensed under CCA-SA 3.0.

Figures 16.2, 16.3 and 16.8 Thinkstock.

Figures 16.4 and 16.5 courtesy Primal Pictures. Used with permission.

Figure 16.6 modified from source image: "Untreated Carpal Tunnel Syndrome" by Dr. Harry Gouvas, MD, PhD. Licensed under Public domain via Wikimedia Commons.

Figures 16.7 and 16.9 courtesy Advanced-Trainings.com.

Study Guide

The Thenar Eminence

1 The text states that the muscles of the thenar eminence have direct connective tissue continuity with _____.

a the carpal trabeculae
b the ulnar nerve
c the flexor retinaculum
d the pronator teres muscle

2 Where does the chapter say that the thumb gets most of its strength and stability from?

a ligaments
b bones
c muscles
d joint capsules

3 According to the text, the symptoms of hand, palm, or wrist pain; with numbness and tingling, are a possible sign of _____.

a muscle hypotonus
b neurovascular compression
c joint dysfunction
d compromised ligaments

4 Compression of which nerve is involved in thenar eminence pain, according to the text?

a ulnar
b median
c radial
d carpal

5 What position should the practitioner's thumbs be in when performing the Thenar Eminence Technique?

a slightly extended
b hyperextended
c slightly flexed
d abducted

For Answer Keys, visit www.Advanced-Trainings.com/v1key/

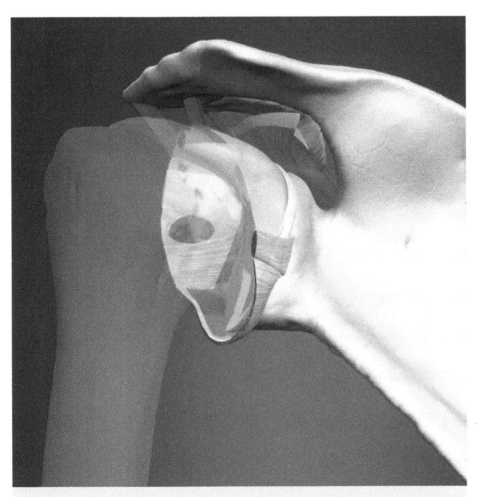

Figure 17.1

The bony socket of the shoulder joint (the glenohumeral fossa) is relatively shallow, getting its stability from the soft tissues of the joint capsule, ligaments (removed in this illustration) and the muscles of the rotator cuff.

The arm needs to move. Reaching, lifting, pulling; hanging, swinging, pushing – the motions of daily life depend on a mobile shoulder. In order to provide the level of mobility the shoulder needs, the bony socket of the shoulder joint (the glenohumeral fossa) is quite shallow. Instead of relying on a deep bony socket like the acetabulum of the hip, the shoulder gets its stability from its soft tissues – the glenohumeral joint capsule and ligaments (Figure 17.1), as well as from the muscles of the rotator cuff. These soft tissue structures allow the necessary balance of stability and movement, yet they are vulnerable to injuries and strain. These result in tissue and tonus changes that can cause these structures to restrict movement, instead of allowing and supporting it.

Sometimes even without an obvious injury, shoulder movement can become quite painful and limited. In these cases, the joint capsule and surrounding facial layers become inflamed and painful, and they can adhere to each other. Idiopathic ("of unknown cause") frozen shoulder (or "adhesive capsulitis", which is the medically preferred term), affects around three percent of the population (1). Though past injury, surgery, or fracture can increase one's likelihood of developing adhesive capsulitis, there are several other non-traumatic risk factors, including being over 40 years old; being female (more than twice as many women as men are affected); prolonged immobility; the presence of heart disease; a diagnosis of Parkinson's; connective tissue maladies; surgery; diabetes; and thyroid issues (in women) (2). There is also speculation that, in some cases, an autoimmune response may be a factor (3).

Within my own practice, my own unscientific observations have been that the majority of those coming with a diagnosis of "frozen shoulder" respond favorably to the techniques described in this chapter (as well as to those presented in the "Rotator Cuff" chapter that follows). In many (if not most) cases, we can reduce pain and achieve greater mobility with our techniques. Often, the changes are rapid, dramatic, and long lasting.

The stubborn minority of cases that do not change significantly seem to be mostly of non-traumatic origin; that is, the shoulder pain and movement limitations arose spontaneously, without apparent injury or a discernible cause (known medically as primary or "genuine" frozen shoulder). Such cases are commonly said to go through three stages: "freezing, painful;" "frozen, stiff;" and "thawing". In my experience, it is the first, most painful stage where the most caution is warranted, as too much work or too direct an approach seems to sometimes aggravate the condition, leading to a painful backlash afterwards. The middle "frozen" stage typically lasts the longest, and seems to be the most challenging to work with, so it is here that our expectations need to be the most modest. The good news is that in most cases, primary frozen shoulder tends to be self-resolving after one to three years, with stretching, hands-on work, and other simple self-care practices showing improvement in recovery times (4).

Even in the minority of clients where shoulder restriction and pain seems impervious to our efforts at direct mobilization, we can often help to ameliorate the side effects and sequelae of shoulder pain and restriction. Frozen shoulder sufferers often experience neck stiffness, headaches, and back pain – all of which can respond positively to our ministrations elsewhere. Unaddressed, these collateral issues can lead to insomnia, depression, and pain fatigue, so it is worthwhile to look for ways to address the issues that come with frozen shoulder, in addition to working with the shoulder itself.

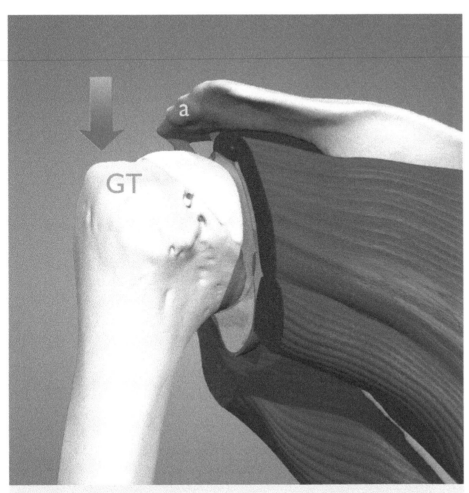

Figure 17.2

Inferior Glide Technique. With palpation, you should feel the greater tuberosity of the humerus (GT) move inferiorly (arrow) with arm abduction. When this inferior glide is lost, the greater tuberosity will ride up to the acromion (a), limiting abduction.

Strategically, I have found the greatest relief if I focus my efforts on restoring glenohumeral abduction, inferior humeral glide, and humeral rotation. In this chapter, I will describe the techniques for restoring these motions.

Inferior Glide of the Humerus Technique

Assessment

Glenohumeral abduction, or bringing the arm out to the side, is often the first movement to show inhibition when the soft tissues of the shoulder joint have lost their elastic mobility. Often, when abduction has been lost, it is linked to a loss of inferior glenohumeral glide.

Try this yourself: raise your arm out to the side while you use your other hand to feel what happens at the greater tuberosity of the humerus, the most lateral bony protuberance of the shoulder. In a healthy shoulder, you will feel this bony prominence drop out from under your touch (move inferiorly) as the arm starts to abduct (Figure 17.2). This is due to the fact that, when unrestricted, the head of the humerus glides inferiorly in the glenohumeral joint as the arm abducts. This inferior motion will be most apparent on the initiation of arm movement – just check the first inch or two (2–5 cm) of movement.

There is a long list of possible soft-tissue contributors to lost inferior glide – shortness or restriction in the deltoid, supraspinatus, or joint capsule; or injury, inflammation, impingement, or adherence of the ligaments, bursa, labrum, or capsule membranes. These most often relate to injuries, posture, and strain, although as discussed above, sometimes there is no apparent cause for a loss of shoulder movement and glide. Whether the cause can be easily determined or not, when inferior humeral glide is lost, the humerus rolls upward in the joint instead of dropping downward. This rolling up causes the greater humeral tuberosity

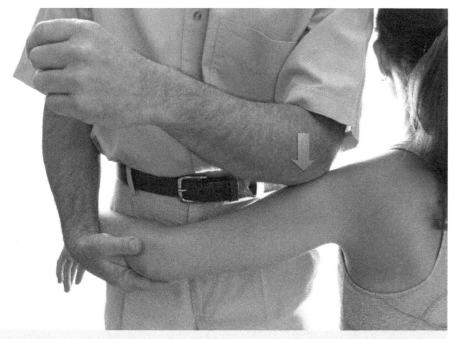

Figure 17.3

Inferior Glide Technique, continued. Use gentle, static pressure with the flat of your ulna, just distal to your elbow, to encourage the greater humeral tuberosity to drop inferiorly when the arm is passively abducted. Check various positions of the arm, waiting in each arm position for an inferior release.

to run into the bony acromion or its ligaments, resulting in discomfort or pain which keeps the arm from rising any further.

It is easiest to assess inferior glide of the humerus with your client sitting up straight on the front edge of a seat. Standing at your client's side, use your thumb to feel for the dropping of the humeral tuberosity with active or passive abduction, as described above. Compare the left and right sides; a side-to-side difference is often more significant than the amount of glide. You will find that a lack of glide on one side frequently corresponds to a loss of abduction and/or glenohumeral pain.

Manipulation

If you find reduced inferior glide of the humerus, you can often improve the range of motion by simply encouraging the head of the humerus to drop inferiorly when the elbow comes out (arm abduction). Use the flat part of your ulna, just in front of (distal to) the point of your elbow, to gently lean on the humerus (Figure 17.3). Without moving your ulna (no sliding, rocking, grinding, and so on), wait for the humerus to respond. Eventually, you will feel it drop slightly in the joint. Move the arm to another position, further forward or back, and repeat, waiting in each place as you feel for the humerus to glide inferiorly. Make sure your pressure does not cause your client discomfort, in the shoulder or elsewhere. Monitor your client's seated position during the work as well – make sure the spine is easy and erect, and the shoulders are square, so that your gentle downward pressure does not collapse your client's seated posture or cause discomfort.

Quite often, this simple technique tangibly improves the shoulder's range of motion and restores the movement options needed for the change to be sustainable. By encouraging inferior glide, you are directly addressing the ligaments and tissues of the joint capsule that can directly contribute to the motion limitations of adhesive capsulitis (5). In other cases, additional work (such as the following "Glenohumeral Capsule Technique") is required.

Key points: Inferior Glide of the Humerus Technique

Indications include:
- Glenohumeral joint pain or movement restrictions, including "Frozen Shoulder"

Purpose
- Assess and restore normal inferior glide of the humerus.

Instructions
1. Feel for the greater tuberosity of the humerus to drop inferiorly with the first 1–2 inches (2–5cm) of glenohumeral abduction.
2. If inferior glide is reduced, mobilize the humerus with direct but sensitive downward pressure to the greater tuberosity, while passively abducting the arm. Do not cause your client pain; wait for myofascial adaptation at positions of restriction or stiff end-feel.
3. Repeat in flexed and extended positions of the glenohumeral joint.

Movements
- Passive abduction of the humerus.

Glenohumeral Capsule Technique

If shoulder motion is still restricted after performing the Inferior Glide technique, the Glenohumeral Capsule Technique can help you get more specific in your work.

With your client in a side-lying position, raise his or her elbow towards the ceiling (passive abduction). While supporting the arm in this abducted position, gently move the forearm, looking for a position where the humerus balances vertically above the glenohumeral joint (Figure 17.4).

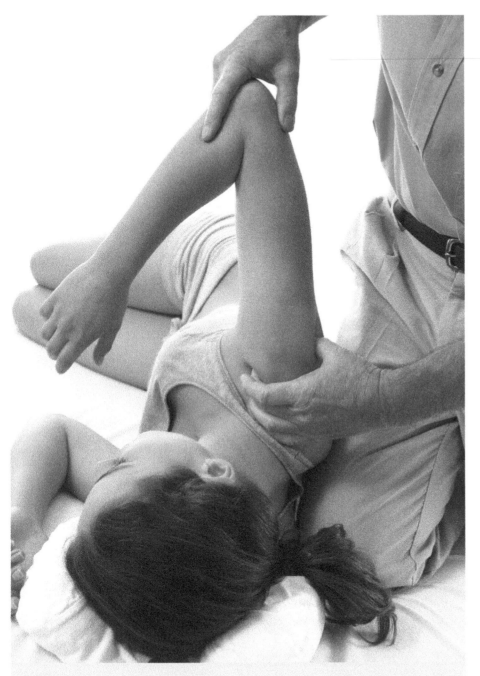

Figure 17.4

In the Glenohumeral Capsule Technique, balance the humerus directly above the scapula, so that passive "swiveling" and "stirring" motions are relatively easy. Use your fingers to feel for soft-tissue restrictions where the humerus articulates with the scapula. Add passive or active humeral rotation, circumduction, and so on, in combination with finger pressure to free up movement and release any restrictions you find.

See video of the Glenohumeral Capsule Technique at http://advanced-trainings.com/v/ab05.html.

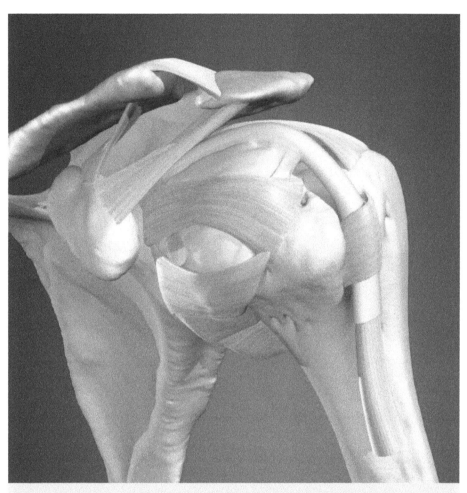

Figure 17.5

The glenohumeral joint capsule's deepest layers are the joint's ligaments and synovial membranes (light blue). Encasing these is a tough sheath of connective tissue (not shown), which forms the outer layer of the capsule. Proximally, these layers blend with the outer edges of the glenoid labrum – the fibrocartilaginous lip of the glenoid fossa.

When you find this balanced position, you can easily use one hand to passively "swivel" (rotate) and "stir" (circumduct) the humerus at the glenohumeral joint.

While moving the arm at the glenohumeral joint, use the fingers and thumb of your other hand to feel around the articulation of the humeral head and the glenoid fossa. With the humerus passively "swiveling" here, you will be able to feel any restrictions in the soft tissues crossing the joint—at the rotator cuff muscles and tendons, the long biceps tendon, the ligaments and tissues of the joint capsule itself (Figure 17.5), and the rotator cuff muscles (Figure 17.6). At their proximal attachments, these ligaments and capsule membranes blend with the outer edges of the labrum, which is the fibrocartilaginous rim that deepens the glenoid fossa. That makes this a useful technique for clients who have been diagnosed with labral tears, or who still have symptoms after labral surgery (once an adequate amount of time has passed for recovery from the surgery itself, of course).

With firm but sensitive finger pressure, search around the joint for thickened, hardened, or immobile tissues. Using your finger pressure, in combination with the movement of the humerus, you can release these areas. In addition to passive movement, you can also use your client's gentle active motions to release any restrictions found.

Hint: be sure to keep your client truly on his or her side, not rolling partly forward or backwards. This makes it easier to find the vertical balance point you need, and it avoids working the shoulder girdle in a protracted or retracted position.

Of course, other structures can contribute to shoulder immobility – for instance, the muscles and fascia of the rotator cuff. In the next chapter, I will discuss ways to assess and work with those important shoulder structures as well.

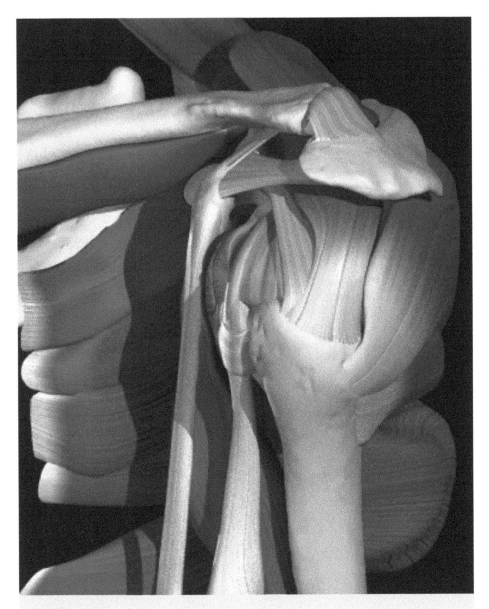

Figure 17.6

The left glenohumeral joint, clavicle, and scapula from a superolateral view. The muscles of the rotator cuff surround the glenohumeral joint capsule. Injuries or strain of these muscles can result in fascial thickening and sensitivity that can be addressed with the Glenohumeral Technique.

Key points: Glenohumeral Capsule Technique

Indications include:

- Glenohumeral joint pain or movement restrictions, including "Frozen Shoulder"
- Rotator cuff pain or movement restriction
- Injury or surgery recovery, once acute phase has passed.

Purpose

- Assess and restore normal adaptability of the glenohumeral joint capsule and ligaments.

Instructions

1. Balance your side-lying client's humerus in a vertical position.
2. Feel for undifferentiated or inelastic tissue around the circumference of the glenohumeral joint capsule, ligaments, labrum, and myofascia of the rotator cuff.
3. Use passive abduction, rotation, and circumduction in combination with your direct pressure to restore differentiation and elasticity to these tissues

Movements

- Passive abduction, rotation, and circumduction of the humerus.

References

[1] Ewald, A. (2011) Adhesive capsulitis: A review. *American Family Physician*. 83(4). p. 417–422, and Pal, B., et al, (1986) Limitation of joint mobility and shoulder capsulitis in insulin- and non-insulin-dependent diabetes mellitus. Br. J. *Rheumatol*. 25. p. 147–151.

[2] Milgrom, C., et al. (2008) Risk factors for idiopathic frozen shoulder. *Isr Med Assoc J*. 10(5). p. 361–364.

[3] Hand, G.C. et al. (2007) The pathology of frozen shoulder. *J Bone Joint Surg Br*. Jul; 89(7) p. 928–32.

[4] Page, P. et al. (2010) Adhesive capsulitis: use the evidence to integrate your interventions. *N Am J Sports Phys Ther*. Dec; 5(4). p. 266–273.

[5] Cochrane, C.G. (1987) Joint mobilization principles: considerations for use in the child with central nervous system dysfunction. *Phys Ther*. 67 p. 1105–1109.

Picture credits

Figures 17.1, 17.2, 17.5 and 17.6 courtesy Primal Pictures. Used with permission.

Figures 17.3 and 17.4 courtesy Advanced-Trainings.com. Used with permission.

Study Guide

Frozen Shoulder, Part 1: The Glenohumeral Joint

1 **Which landmark is used to assess inferior glide of the humerus (as described in the text)?**

a the acromion process
b lateral head of the clavicle
c greater tubercle of the humerus
d the spine of the scapula

2 **What is the practitioner feeling for in the assessment phase of the Inferior Glenohumeral Glide Technique?**

a amount of glide
b side to side comparison
c presence of crepitus
d loss of glenohumeral adduction

3 **What does the text suggest doing once the practitioner feels the humerus drop in the Inferior Glide Technique?**

a put the arm down
b assess the other side
c move the arm into another position
d wait for the humerus to drop some more

4 **What does the text state that the practitioner is feeling for in the Glenohumeral Capsule Technique?**

a joint clicking or popping
b the inferior glide of the humerus
c soft tissue restrictions
d restricted scapular movement

5 **What does the text state that the proximal glenohumeral ligaments and joint capsule blend with?**

a the rotator cuff muscles
b the labrum
c the sternum
d the greater tuberosity

For Answer Keys, visit www.Advanced-Trainings.com/v1key/

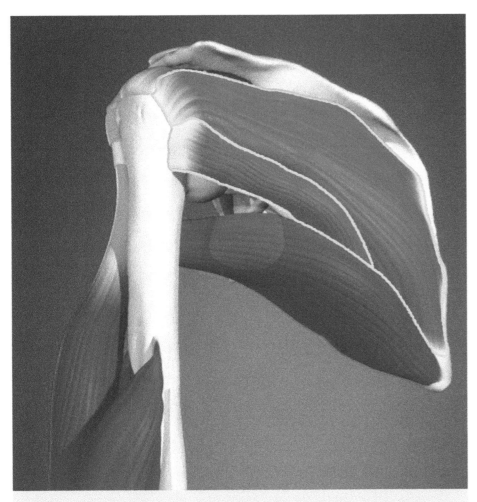

Figure 18.1

The posterior aspect of the rotator cuff includes the infraspinatus and teres minor muscles (in orange). Together with the other muscles of the rotator cuff, these structures play key roles in glenohumeral joint mobility and balance. The circular subtendinous bursa of the teres major is faintly visible in this view and can be tender when worked.

In the previous chapter, we looked at ways to assess and restore the crucial movement of inferior glide of the humerus (in a healthy shoulder, the head of the humerus drops inferiorly as it begins abduction). The two additional techniques described in this chapter will give you more ways to regain lost inferior humeral glide and to address rotation restrictions – two of the motions that are often restricted in "frozen shoulder" or adhesive capsulitis (1). Additionally, since these techniques work with front/back balance of key structures surrounding the glenohumeral joint (GHJ), they are also indicated when you see a postural tendency towards either internal or external arm rotation at the GHJ (described below).

Posterior Rotator Cuff Technique

Work with the posterior side of the rotator cuff is indicated when:

- the arm's resting position tends towards external rotation
- internal rotation is limited or painful, or
- arm abduction is limited (as in Figure 18.7 on page 223).

Position your prone client so that his or her arm hangs off the side of the table, with the table's edge positioned directly below (anterior to) the GHJ. In this way, gravity and the edge of the table help open up the posterior side of the rotator cuff (Figure 18.1). With some tables, you will need to add a folded towel or other additional padding over the table's edge so that it is comfortable for your client.

With the arm hanging off the edge of the table, work the muscles and fasciae on the posterior side of the scapula with the knuckles of your soft, open fist (Figure 18.2). Generally, a lateral

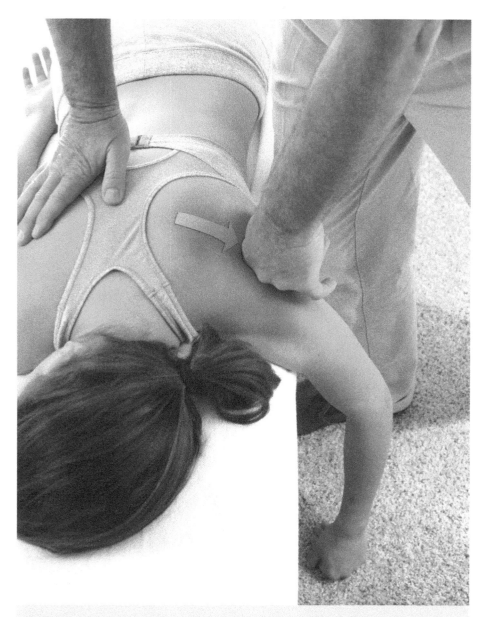

Figure 18.2
Posterior Rotator Cuff Technique. With your client's arm hanging, use the knuckles of a soft fist or another tool to release any restrictions between the humerus and scapula. Active client movements can include arm rotation, extension, or reaching overhead.

direction to your work will be most effective. Make sure your pressure is comfortable for your client. Feel for differentiation and increased elasticity in the infraspinatus, teres major and minor, posterior deltoid, and their respective fascias. If you have observed restricted abduction or reduced inferior glenohumeral glide (as discussed above), be sure to work the supraspinatus muscle along the superior margin of the scapula – it plays an important role in these motions.

Your client can assist the release by gently and slowly swiveling his or her arm (active rotation of the humerus) while continuing to let the arm hang. Other movement variations include slow, active glenohumeral circumduction, as well as asking the client to gently reach overhead (glenohumeral flexion). When using these movements, you can change the direction of your pressure from lateral to medial, so as to encourage the soft tissue of the posterior scapula to release medially and inferiorly (away from the direction of the reach).

All active movements should be slow and gentle enough that the muscle's contraction does not push you out of the tissues that you are working. Coach your client to use just the initiation of hand or arm movement – only the first few millimeters – as this can make this way of initiating movement clearer for both of you. Ask your client to begin the movements very gradually, reaching first with just the hand, and then just the hand and forearm, before engaging the shoulder muscles at all.

On clients who are larger than you are, you may find that there is an advantage in gently using your forearm (not the point of the elbow) in place of the soft fist. Work slowly and sensitively here; the axillary and suprascapular nerves are in this area, as is a bursa between the tendons of the triceps' long head and the teres major (Figure 18.1). All of these structures can be quite tender; in addition, the forearm is a powerful tool.

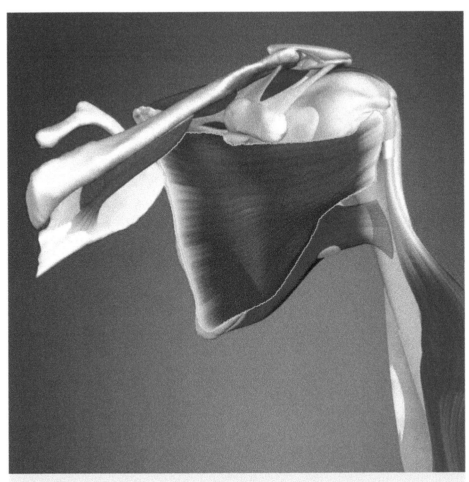

Figure 18.3

Covering the entire anterior side of the scapula, the subscapularis (green) is the largest and strongest of the shoulder rotators.

Indications include:
- Glenohumeral joint pain or movement restrictions, including "frozen shoulder," shoulder impingement syndrome, recovery from injury and surgery, etc.
- Externally rotated position of the arm in its resting position.

Purpose
- Restore normal range of glenohumeral abduction, flexion, and rotation.

Instructions
1. With client's arm hanging off the edge of the table, work the myofascial structures on the posterior side of the scapula, using the knuckles of a soft fist.
2. Coach your client to initiate active movements slowly enough so that you aren't pushed out of the muscle. Work with slow, smooth initiation of movement.

Movements
- Slow, small active movements of the hanging arm, in all directions: reaching overhead, rotation while hanging, abduction, etc.

Subscapularis Technique

See video of the Subscapularis Technique at http://advanced-trainings.com/v/ab06.html.

Once you have thoroughly addressed the posterior side of the rotator cuff with the previous technique, you will want to balance the shoulder girdle by working the front side of the GHJ as well. The subscapularis is a good place to start, as it is the deepest muscle on the anterior side of the GHJ (Figures 18.3 and 18.4). In addition, it is the largest and strongest of the rotator cuff muscles. Since the subscapularis and its tendon are implicated in many rotator cuff tears, in some cases of shoulder impingement, as well as in chronically dislocating shoulders, it is often affected by the surgical interventions that are used for these conditions. Loss of tissue elasticity and adhesions after surgery are the main causes for re-injury (2).

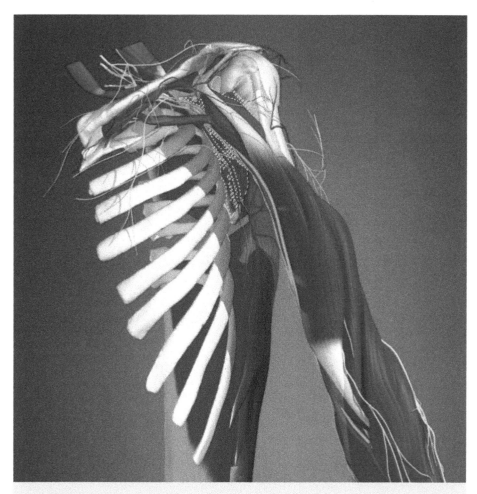

Figure 18.4

The subscapularis (green) is sandwiched between the shoulder blade and the ribcage, forming much of the posterior wall of the axillary space.

The subscapularis also plays a direct role in regulating inferior humeral glide. Rather than allowing the abducting humerus to rock upwards on the fossa (like the rockers of a rocking chair would move on the floor), the subscapularis helps centralize the humeral head in the fossa, causing the humerus to glide rather than roll in the fossa. This is helpful, but if the subscapularis is too active, tight, or shortened, it will inhibit abduction (as well as external rotation).

There are several ways to work the subscapularis, but one of the least invasive and most effective methods is pictured in Figure 18.5. From behind your side-lying client, cradle his or her arm in the crook of your elbow, and with this same arm, lay your hand palm-down on the ribs of the axillary space. Although this will be your "working" hand, it stays relatively soft and relaxed, using no more effort or stiffness than necessary. With your other hand behind the shoulder, roll the scapula over this working hand, so that the tips and lateral edges of fingers of your anterior, working hand can feel the subscapularis on the anterior side of the scapula. The skin, lymph structures, and nerves of the axillary region (Figure 18.4) are particularly delicate, so do not poke, chisel, or force your fingers in. Wait for your client's breath and relaxation to open up the space between the scapula and the ribcage to allow you to reach the anterior side of the scapula.

Once you have arrived at the scapula, you can ask your client to do slight movements of arm abduction or rotation. This muscle activation will allow you to feel the subscapularis and be even more specific with your work. However, do not ask for so much movement that the scapula clamps back down on the ribcage. Encourage your client to let the subscapular space become as easy and open as possible, even when performing the active movements of the arm. Work as much of the front side of the scapula as you

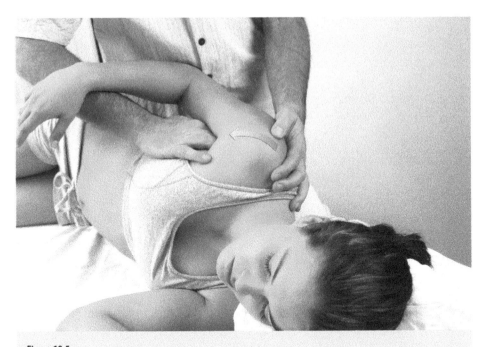

Figure 18.5

In the Subscapularis Technique, cradle your client's arm and shoulder complex from front and back. Use your posterior hand to "feed" the scapula over the fingers of your anterior hand, which is then in position to delicately work the subscapularis with your fingertips, while your client plays with gentle arm abduction and rotation.

can comfortably reach, especially since the subscapularis is a large muscle, covering most of the anterior scapula.

Key points: Subscapularis Technique

Indications include:
- Rotator cuff pain or movement restriction;
- Internally rotated position of the arm in its resting position.

Purpose
- Restore normal range of glenohumeral abduction and external rotation;
- Balance the posterior-side work of the previous Posterior Rotator Cuff Technique.

Instructions
- Gently roll (protract) the scapula over a hand placed on the ribcage. Use the tips and lateral edges of your fingers to work the subscapularis on the anterior side of the scapula.

Movements
- Breath
- Slow, active abduction, rotation, flexion, and extension of the glenohumeral joint.

Cautions
- Use care working near the delicate skin, lymph nodes, nerves, and tissues of the axilla.

Putting it together

Is the ordering of the Posterior Rotator Cuff and the Subscapularis Techniques important? Given their front/back relationship to the humerus (Figure 18.6), these two techniques have complementary effects on arm rotation. Since we are working with our client's proprioception, as well as any tissues, the way we sequence our techniques can emphasize particular aspects of the work in our client's proprioceptive awareness.

For example, probably the most common shoulder pattern is the tendency towards

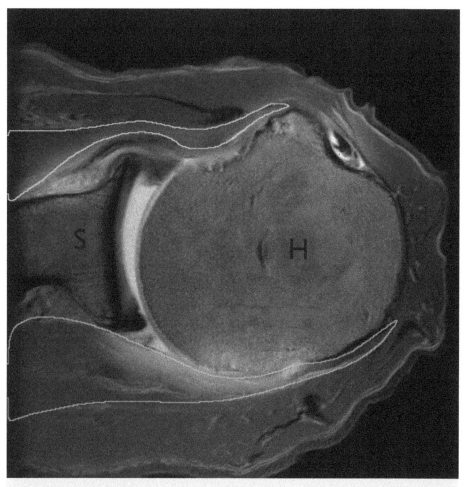

Figure 18.6

Axial (horizontal) cross-section MRI of the head of the humerus and rotator cuff. The subscapularis (outlined in green) on the anterior side of the shoulder, and the infraspinatus (orange) on the posterior side work together to coordinate rotation of the humerus (H) in relation to the scapula (S).

forward-rounding the shoulders. Key elements of this pattern are the rounded posture of scapular protraction on the ribcage; the elbow of the hanging arm pointing out to the side; and greater resistance to passive external humeral rotation. In this case, most people will feel greater balance and ease if you end your work on a note of anterior release by working the subscapularis after working the posterior rotator cuff.

In contrast, chronic external rotation of the humerus is most often associated with the "pulled-back" posture of shoulder retraction, and the elbow points more posteriorly, or even posteromedially. Switch the order of these techniques in this case, so as to finish with a sense of openness across the posterior side of the shoulders and back. You will also see clients who have more internal humeral rotation on one side, and more external rotation on the other side, especially when there is a larger asymmetrical pattern, such as with spinal scoliosis. In these cases, use different ordering on each side, ending with work on the shorter aspect.

Of course with both internal and external shoulder patterns, there can be many other structures involved in addition to those discussed here. In internal rotation patterns, look for involvement of the pectoralis major, pectoralis minor, and anterior thoracic fasciae, as well as exhalation-dominant breathing and rib patterns. In externally rotated patterns, you may need to address the trapezius, rhomboids, and serratus posterior superior, which are the larger structures of the back. Inhalation-dominant breathing, diaphragm, and ribcage patterns can also contribute to the tendency towards external rotation in the upper limb. In both internal and external patterns, pelvis resting position and spinal curves can play a large part as well.

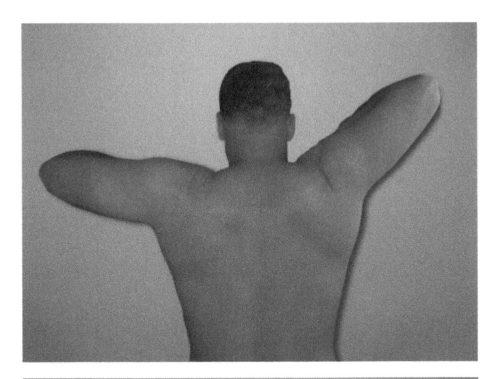

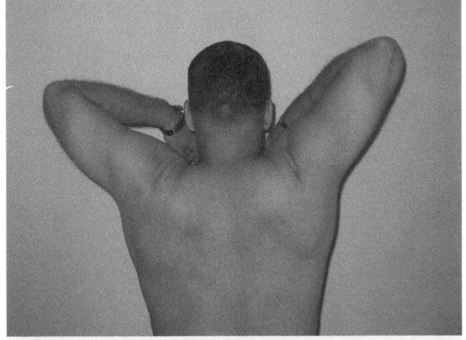

Figures 18.7/18.8

A client with rotator cuff pain and restriction shows improved abduction as a result of increased inferior glide of the humerus. Photos were taken before and after two sessions of myofascial work, employing the techniques described here.

Visual case study

The before-and-after photos of the client in Figures 18.7 and 18.8 show significant range of motion increases after two sessions utilizing the myofascial techniques described in this and the previous chapters. The client underwent rotator cuff surgery for pain and restriction in his left shoulder (probably related to weightlifting), about two years before coming to my practice for myofascial work. His range of motion limitations and pain had continued after surgery, but they improved substantially after receiving myofascial work. His range of motion continued to improve after the photos were taken, and several years later, he is quite physically active and pain free, and continues to come for less frequent "maintenance" sessions.

As with other conditions, continuing unexplained pain or pronounced movement restrictions can be cause for referral to a physician or orthopedic specialist. And while not all clients respond as dramatically as the example described above, this amount of improvement is not unusual. You will find that the concepts and techniques described in this chapter, as well as those addressed in the previous chapter, will benefit a very large number of your clients who experience shoulder restriction and pain.

References

[1] Kapandji, I.A. (1982). *The Physiology of the Joints: Volume One Upper Limb* (5th ed.). New York, NY: Churchill Livingstone. p. 30.
[2] Bartl, C. et al. (2012) Long-term outcome and structural integrity following open repair of massive rotator cuff tears. *Int J Shoulder Surg.* 6. p. 1–8.

Picture credits

Figures 18.1, 18.3, 18.4 and 18.6 courtesy Primal Pictures. Used with permission.
Figures 18.2, 18.5, 18.7 and 18.8 courtesy Advanced-Trainings.com.

Study Guide

Frozen Shoulder, Part 2: The Rotator Cuff

1 In the Posterior Rotator Cuff Technique, what is the suggested direction of pressure in combination with the client's active movement?

a medially and inferiorly
b laterally
c superiorly
d medially and superiorly

2 What is the suggested movement cue for initiating active movement in the Posterior Rotator Cuff Technique?

a start with shoulder movements
b start with forearm movements
c start with elbow movements
d start with hand movements

3 How does the text describe the subscapularis' role in coordinating glenohumeral glide?

a initiates internal rotation of the humerus
b prevents external rotation of the humerus
c centralizes humeral head
d stabilizes the olecranon

4 As described in the text, what does the practitioner's posterior hand do in the Subscapularis Technique?

a feels for restrictions around the rotator cuff
b glides under the posterior scapula
c helps fold the anterior scapula onto the front hand
d applies inferior pressure to the scapula

5 As stated in the text, in combination with what motion does a healthy shoulder drop inferiorly?

a external humeral rotation
b glenohumeral adduction
c internal humeral rotation
d glenohumeral abduction

For Answer Keys, visit www.Advanced-Trainings.com/v1key/

Index

Note: Page number followed by 'f' indicates figure only.